EATING FOR ACID REFLUX

E A T I N G   F O R

ACID REFLUX

A Handbook and Cookbook for Those with Heartburn

JILL SKLAR and ANNABEL COHEN

Foreword by Manuel Sklar, M.D.

Da Capo
LIFE
LONG

A MEMBER OF THE PERSEUS BOOKS GROUP

Cataloging-in-Publication data for this book is available from the Library of Congress.

ISBN-13: 978-1-56924-492-0

Published by Da Capo Press
A Member of the Perseus Books Group
www.dacapopress.com
Note: The information in this book is true and complete to the best of our knowledge. This book is intended only as an informative guide for those wishing to know more about health issues. In no way is this book intended to replace, countermand, or conflict with the advice given to you by your own physician. The ultimate decision concerning care should be made between you and your doctor. We strongly recommend you follow his or her advice. Information in this book is general and is offered with no guarantees on the part of the authors or Da Capo Press. The authors and publisher disclaim all liability in connection with the use of this book. The names and identifying details of people associated with events described in this book have been changed. Any similarity to actual persons is coincidental.

Da Capo Press books are available at special discounts for bulk purchases in the U.S. by corporations, institutions, and other organizations. For more information, please contact the Special Markets Department at the Perseus Books Group, 2300 Chestnut Street, Suite 200, Philadelphia, PA, 19103, or call (800) 255-1514, or e-mail special.markets@perseusbooks.com.

10 9

To Joel and Jonah, who are my two great loves;
To my sister, Patrice, who astonishes me with her grace and bravery;
To my brother, Eric, whose loyalty is unending;
To my mother, Kathryn, who first taught me to love.
—Jill Sklar

To Raquel, my raison d'etre *and my parents,*
for whom I only wish long and healthy lives.
—Annabel Cohen

CONTENTS

FOREWORD

By Manuel Sklar, M.D.

It is the rare person who has not experienced heartburn. For many, an occasional antacid will do, but for others, expensive medications to be taken on a daily basis, often for an indefinite time, may be necessary. A few may even require surgical management. This condition is called gastroesophageal reflux disease (GERD), an acid aggressive disorder caused by malfunction of the lower esophageal sphincter allowing acid to flow into the esophagus causing irritation and often inflammation of the esophageal lining. This disorder has important implications because of its detrimental effect on the quality of life and the relationship to esophageal cancer, an increasing and life-threatening problem often preceded by premalignant change in the esophageal mucosa known as Barrett's esophagus.

The authors, Jill Sklar and Annabel Cohen, have thoughtfully and thoroughly covered virtually ever aspect of this disease. The initial chapters are devoted to a description of the typical and atypical features of the clinical picture such as the type and nature of pain and the consequences of regurgitation; heartburn (more technically known as pyrosis), cough, asthma, and laryngeal symptoms. The pathophysiology of reflux is then described in great detail in regard to the abnormal function of the lower esophageal segment, the importance of hiatus hernia, and the effects of acid. The methods of diagnosis are elaborated, including radiological studies, endoscopic procedures, motility studies, and, the gold standard of establishing GERD, the 24-hour pH monitoring. The methodology and role of each of these tests are explained from the patient's viewpoint. Treatment is then discussed and virtually every pharmacologic modality is covered, including antacids, H_2 blockers, proton pump inhibitors, and promotility drugs. The value and side effects of each of these drug classes are delineated. The management of complications such as stricture, failure of medical therapy, and indications for surgery is next considered. A description of the various surgical procedures, including the various types of fundoplasty, open and laparoscopic, as well as the newest endoscopic techniques is offered. Special attention is given to the problem of Barrett's esophagus, including surveillance and ways of dealing with dysplasia. The clinical portion then concludes with several interesting subjects. One deals with alternative medical approaches to GERD. Heartburn in pregnancy is next covered in great detail with many novel ideas for control, and finally the unique presentation and treatment of GERD in children and in the elderly are considered. The last chapter deals with lifestyle modification. These include practical suggestions regarding appropriate diet, optimal timing of meals, postural alteration, and the importance of weight loss, avoidance of alcohol, and smoking cessation.

The most unusual feature of the book and one of its highlights is the presentation of over one hundred recipes designed to be suitable for the GERD sufferer. Basically, these foods are low in fat and sugar as well as low acidic, but high in flavor and variety. I am quite certain that they will be most welcome by the GERD patient and add to the quality of life.

MANUEL SKLAR, M.D., F.A.C.S., F.A.C.G., is Chief, Section of Gastroenterology, Sinai-Grace Hospital, and Clinical Professor of Medicine at Wayne State University School of Medicine. He lives in Franklin, Michigan.

PART 1

THE HANDBOOK

Introduction

Reflux discovered my brother, my sister, and me nearly simultaneously within the past seven years.

My sister, Patrice, the eldest of us three, was the first to experience the condition as she weathered occasional bouts during several months of two pregnancies. During this time, she learned a few tricks of the trade, like propping herself up with pillows as she slept or avoiding bending from the waist. But it wasn't until a few years later, in 1995, when she awoke from her sleep with a searing pain in her chest and a nagging feeling that this was nothing to ignore. For days and months afterward, she would prop herself up in an effort to stay awake until the pain either subsided or killed her.

"It was really scary. I didn't tell anyone," she said.

She finally caved in one day and headed for the emergency room. There, doctors ran every conceivable cardiac test and came up with nothing but a bill for $1,700 and advice to take over-the-counter pain medication. Her internist took more of an interest. He wanted to know if the pain occurred when she was lying down? Did it happen sometimes after meals? When she bent down after eating, did a sour taste fill her palate? She answered yes to all of the questions. He told Patrice it was likely to be reflux and handed her a prescription for an acid reducer.

Shortly after Patrice was diagnosed, my little brother, Eric, began to have problems as well. First, he noticed that he had this dry little cough, not very annoying but noticeable enough that it bugged him. Then, he kept waking up in the morning with a sore throat. Time after time, the symptom would go away during the day only to return next morning. Next, his voice became hoarse, a sound that began to follow him through the day. Sleep escaped him as burning pains often woke him up in the middle of the night. Fairly keen about change in his health, he decided to go to the doctor, just to be on the safe side.

The internist said it was probably just a virus or a bug, prescribed an antibiotic, and sent him away. A friend, a speech pathologist by training, noticed a change in Eric's voice and told him to have it checked out by an ear, nose, and throat specialist. After an endoscopic exam, the specialist concurred, saying his vocal cords had been damaged by the reflux. He was given a prescription of Prevacid, a medication that cleared up all of his symptoms.

Then, it was my turn. Approaching the third trimester of my pregnancy, I began to notice a sense of nausea after I ate, followed by what I can best describe as sour burps. At night, the situation worsened, robbing me of sleep when burning pains in my mid-chest kept me awake. I begged my obstetrician for some relief, and he told me to take an antacid and avoid spicy foods. I gave up barbecued ribs and chicken, spicy hot peppers, tomatoes and anything made with them, chocolate, and my mom's onion soup. Despite following his advice, the condition seemed to worsen. I called Patrice, who told me about raising the head of my bed. When I asked her what she could eat without pain, the answer was bleak. "You want to know the diet for reflux? It is a plain baked potato, no butter, no sour cream, and no pepper," she said.

Not long after my symptoms subsided, Annabel began to notice something strange happening to her. First, she could only sleep sitting up as chest pain would jolt her awake when she reclined flat. Next, she got a cough and a sore throat that she couldn't shake. Then foods began to bother her, even when she was awake, a tough situation as she makes part of her living as a food writer and chef. "I eliminated whole categories of foods from my diet."

She finally went for help when fears of a heart condition began to haunt her. Now, through medication and diet modification, she is able to fend off the effects of reflux.

More and more people began to share their stories with Annabel and me as they learned we were writing this book. One friend slept on a stack of pillows, an economy-sized jar of Rolaids on her bedside table. Another shared a tale of waking in the middle of the night to intense searing pain, immediately regretting his ritual of a scotch before nodding off. A high school friend told me his daughter had horrendous reflux that was treated only through medication and tilting her mattress at night. A man I interviewed for a story reported losing twenty pounds, mostly due to not being able to tolerate his usual diet. At a dinner party Annabel threw, nearly all of the guests shared either a personal story about struggling with the condition or one of someone close to them. All of them had to alter their diet and lifestyle, consequently feeling deprived in doing so.

I could go on and on with all of the stories I have collected from people but the message is always the same. There is pain, there is diagnosis, and then there is treatment with medication and, at times, surgery. Patients sometimes have little information about lifestyle changes that can be made to lessen the scope of the condition. Without treatment, the condition can advance the damage to a point where the conditions are ripe for the formation of esophageal cancer, usually a deadly disease.

The more I talked to people about the condition, the more I realized that there was a need for a book like this one, one that combined medical information, tips for living from people struggling daily with the disease, and recipes made from ingredients that do not promote symptoms yet are tasty and nutritious.

How to use this book

THE BOOK YOU have in your hands is a handbook and a cookbook, all in one. It is designed for use for all of those who have reflux, from the newly diagnosed to the old pros and everyone in between.

The pages in the front of the book are designed to walk the reader—presumably a patient or a friend or family member—through the various medical and surgical treatment options, alternative treatments, and lifestyle modifications that can be made to ease the symptoms of and damage caused by acid reflux. What you will not find in the front part of the book is a prescription for treatment; I am a medical writer, not a doctor. The point of the book is to educate the reader about the disease and its treatments, allowing her to make informed decisions about her course of action and to become her best advocate in medical matters relating to reflux.

The book opens by painting an epidemiological picture of the disease. It then explains the basics of human digestion and what goes wrong to cause the symptoms of reflux. It follows a patient through the diagnostic process, explaining the tests and how other diseases and disorders are ruled out.

A reader may find great value in the portion of the book dedicated to lifestyle modification. By making simple adjustments in the area of diet, sleeping conditions, exercise, weight loss, smoking cessation, and clothing, many people with reflux find relief from many of their symptoms. Particularly changing what, when, and how you consume foods can have great bearing on reducing the effects of acid reflux. In fact, doctors often suggest these changes at the first sign of the condition.

The book then addresses the various medical treatment options available for reflux patients and when those treatments are best utilized; it also discusses medications for other conditions that can potentially exacerbate the condition. For surgery, the options are fully explained and a guide to the hospital experience is offered. Alternative treatments—everything from aloe vera juice to yoga—are highlighted to suit those who prefer these complementary treatments. How these different approaches affect the young, the pregnant, and the elderly also are discussed.

That leads us to the second half of the book, an extensive collection of recipes for individuals who find that a low-fat, low-acid diet can ease the burning pain of reflux. The recipes were created by Annabel, my writing partner as well as a reflux patient and an experienced chef, and have been tested in regular kitchens by real reflux patients just like you. Every food category that would appear in a regular cookbook appears here, from appetizers to desserts, beverages to soups and everything in between. And those comfort foods you thought you could no longer eat—think fried chicken and mashed potatoes—have been adapted to have the same great taste but less fat. The same goes for those ethnic dishes you find in Italian, Mexican, and Thai restaurants that you thought you could no longer consume without practically keeling over.

And the great thing about the recipes is that everyone can make them, from the novice chef to the most discriminating foodie. They are easy to make and delicious, lending themselves to elegant presentations for elaborate dinner parties or for every-day food you can share with your family. They taste so good that your family and friends won't miss out on the things that would make you miserable—the stomach-slowing fat and the pain-inducing acid.

Following the cookbook, a resource guide will point out the best books you can buy on the subject of reflux as well as places you can find information and support. A glossary also explains some of the more technical terms highlighted in the earlier text—words that appear in boldface in the text appear in the glossary.

NOT THE END OF THE WORLD

THROUGH THE USE OF this book, Annabel and I hope you will learn that having reflux is not the end of the world, that it is manageable with medication, surgery, and lifestyle modification, including diet. Hopefully, the condition will go from the thing that keeps you up at night to the thing you barely remember that you have. You can—and should—lead a fulfilling life, with or without reflux.

—*Jill Sklar*

1

WHY *NOT* YOU?

M AYBE YOU HAVE suspected this news was coming all along and so hearing that you have **gastroesophageal reflux disease (GERD)** is not such a big deal. Perhaps you really thought that you were dying of something drastic like cancer or had a serious cardiac experience such as a heart attack so the news is actually a huge and welcome relief. For others, you may have lived a life without anything more serious than the stomach flu, so finding out that you have a disease can be a significant letdown, leaving you to utter the often-asked question, "Why me?"

Whatever the case, you now have joined a club with literally millions of other members worldwide. Simply based on the odds, it is fairly likely that you or someone you love will experience this illness at some point or another. In fact, your odds of developing reflux are greater than developing any other gastrointestinal condition, save viral or bacterial infection resulting in diarrhea or vomiting. That is not exactly a soothing reality. Still, though you probably never wanted to be a part of the club, there are certainly worse ones to join.

The important thing to realize now is that you are doing something about the situation. By learning about the symptoms of, causes for, and treatments of the disease, you are equipping yourself with a knowledge that likely will make you a better partner in finding your own solutions to the challenges you face as a result of the disease, thus allowing you to continue to lead a normal life.

What is GERD?

WE WILL GET into a complete description of the process of GERD in the next chapter, but for now, a little bit of a definition of the condition is required here. Call it **reflux, acid reflux, heartburn,** or GERD, it is essentially the same thing and you have it. The normal process begins when food, after being chewed and swallowed, enters the **stomach**. There, it must be broken down rather extensively for the nutrients to be absorbed in the small intestine. Not relying on muscular action alone, the stomach produces **enzymes** and gastric juices, principally **hydrochloric acid** and **pepsin,** to help break down the food. During normal digestion, a **sphincter** that demarcates the border between the **esophagus** and the stomach, the **lower esophageal sphincter** or **LES,** remains closed in order to prevent the digested food from migrating in the wrong direction.

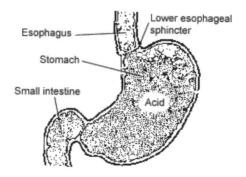

Figure 1. Lower Esophageal Sphincter

Source: *Digestive Disease Dictionary,* a publication of the National Institute for Diabetes, Digestive and Kidney Diseases

But in reflux, the dynamic changes. Either as the food is being digested or after it has left the stomach, the excess acid splashes past a weakened, inhibited, or malfunctioning LES. This sphincter can lose its tension for a variety of reasons but the effect is pretty much the same: the acid and pepsin travel up the esophagus, irritating the sensitive innermost lining of the esophagus, the **mucosa,** which is not able to withstand the erosive qualities of these liquids.

Briefly, the backwashing digestive juices can cause quite a bit of damage over time, leaving erosions, inflammation, and, at times, scar tissue on the mucosa; at its worst, the prolonged damage by the acid and pepsin is a known and prominent cause for **esophageal cancer**, a disease that is diagnosed in more than 13,000 Americans each year and leads to the deaths of 12,600 more, according to the American Cancer Society's 2002 statistics.

GERD manifests itself in different ways. Perhaps you started out with nothing more than a sore throat or a husky voice. That is not unusual. Others are awakened by chest pain that resembles a heart attack; some feel a stabbing or burning pain in their chest or feel lightheaded or faint; many have persistent coughing, clearing of the throat, or asthma-like symptoms, such as laboring to breathe due to acid that has been aspirated; and still more experience the acrid taste of the acid, the same substance that a builder often uses to clean concrete, as it creeps into their mouths.

In the following chapters, we will get into the pathophysiology (the alteration of normal bodily function as seen in diseases) of GERD and examine the different paths you can take toward recovery and maintenance. But for now, it is really important for you to realize that you are not alone in this.

THE HISTORY OF GERD

FOR MILLENNIA, PEOPLE have suffered with the symptoms of heartburn. Evidence of early treatments for the disease includes a variety of treatments that were used historically to treat it in different cultures. For example, the Malawi tribe in Africa boiled the root of the jasmine plant to soothe heartburn while the ancient midwives of different cultures doled out ginger, coriander, and cilantro for their patients to chew on when they experienced pregnancy-related heartburn.

But it was difficult to actually find the cause of the disease since there were no ways of personally witnessing not only exactly how digestion worked but also what the physical manifestations of the disease included. The esophagus of an adult is approximately nine inches long (give or take an inch or two for an adjustment for overall height), too long for a primitively equipped physician to examine.

In fact, digestion itself was poorly understood until recent times. Ancient peoples had different ideas about what took place after food was swallowed. Some believed that an internal combustion—a "fire in the belly"—occurred, not much different from the type of fire over which their food was cooked. Others believed it was solely the mechanical action of the stomach that broke down food for digestion. Doctors often theorized about the ways and means of digestion and even experimented on themselves and others to prove their ideas.

Knowledge took a big leap forward when a young man named Alexis St. Mornay was accidentally shot in the stomach while standing in the small front room of the fur trading company of John Jacob Astor on Mackinac Island, a small splash of land in the strait between the northern and southern peninsulas that make up the state of Michigan. Lucky for young Alexis, the small wooden trading company building was located within spitting distance of Fort Mackinac, an American military installation that was staffed by Dr. William Beaumont. St. Mornay survived the initial shot but the wound never completely healed and formed a gastric fistula, a tunnel-like opening between the skin and the stomach. In the next several years, Dr. Beaumont was able to learn exactly how food was digested by peering into the hole, putting things into it, and suctioning things out of it. He conducted many experiments on this patient over the years; for example, Dr. Beaumont inserted bits of meat securely fastened to strings into the man's stomach opening, withdrawing them occasionally to see what was left of the meat. From this research, we learned about the gastric juices and other valuable tidbits, such as how long it takes for a piece of beef to digest (approximately four hours, in case you were wondering). A fascinating interactive educational monument to Dr. Beaumont and his findings remains on what is now a beautiful resort island.

But it took another several decades for the knowledge about reflux to take another step forward. Surprisingly, it wasn't until electric lights were created and refined that the world of **endoscopy** was created. This advance meant that doctors were able to literally shine a light on previously unexplored regions of the living human body. At first, the instruments were used to examine the rectum, using a series of mirrors to reflect back images. Later, scopes incorporated other emerging technology such as biopsy snares to extract tissue samples and fiberoptic lighting and imaging to allow the doctor to view the inside of the curvy GI tract, inventions that make endoscopy a lot more tolerable and useful than the original rigid and limited tools.

But to simply see a disease process was not enough. Identification of abnormal structures and functions led to theorizing as to why and how these manifestations occurred. In his seminal work, *The Growth of Gastroenterologic Knowledge during the Twentieth Century*, Dr. Joseph Kirsner pinpoints the exact time at which it was suspected that the hydrochloric acid and pepsin secreted by the stomach caused the erosive lesions on the esophagi of several patients. In a scientific paper published in the *Journal of the American Medical Association* in 1935, a doctor theorized that these lesions seen in five patients were actually "peptic esophagitis" that resulted from the backwash of the gastric juices. In a different journal eleven years later, the disease was tagged as "reflux esophagitis."

In the ensuing years, many scientists were eager to find a cause for this condition, many of whom tried to label **hiatal hernia**, a condition in which the upper part of the stomach pushes up through the diaphragm, as the chief culprit; however, sometimes the disease occurred in the absence of such a condition. It wasn't until the late 1960s and early 1970s that a malfunctioning LES was nabbed as another suspect.

Since that time, a number of medical and surgical approaches to treating the disease have been developed. Some have shown early promise only to be discarded with the creation of new and different treatments; others have remained a mainstay for the more mildly affected. In that vein, more and more doctors and scientists continue to work on the cause, issuing studies and case reports nearly every month. And as they do so, diagnosis methods and treatments will continue to evolve.

THE EPIDEMIOLOGY OF GERD

ALL AROUND THE world, scientists known as epidemiologists study the occurrence of certain aspects of health and well-being in different areas in an effort to track disease patterns in a variety of cultures. They look into, for example, heart disease patterns in a certain area, the quantity and quality of the food and drink inhabitants consume, whether they smoke, what kinds of exercise they get and how often they get it. Information from studies like this led scientists to believe that the Mediterranean diet was good for heart health while the common American diet was not as beneficial. From this information, the scientists are able to grasp how certain factors and conditions can impact health. For reflux, this is no different. Epidemiologists have learned a number of things about who develops reflux, where it occurs, and how often it happens.

Studies vary in the percentage of Americans who have GERD. One often quoted, albeit dated, study found that 7 percent of the population experienced daily heartburn with another 36 percent complaining of nightly symptoms (Nebel, O.T., et al., *American Journal of Digestive Disorders* 1976; 21:953–956). That study also found little difference in the age or gender of the sufferers, with the exception of pregnant women, 25 percent of whom reported daily symptoms and 52 percent of whom reported monthly symptoms. The American Gastroenterological Association (AGA) puts the figure in round numbers at 60 million adults who experience it at least once a month while 25 million of those have daily pain due to the condition; a Gallup poll conducted in 2000 with the AGA found that 80 percent of those with heartburn or approximately 50 million Americans experienced nighttime symptoms.

In other developed countries, the numbers are strikingly similar. A study found that 25 percent of Swedes suffered GERD-related problems with 21 percent having heartburn, 20 percent experiencing acid regurgitation, and 12 percent having non-cardiac chest pain (Ruth, M., et al., *Scandinavian Journal of Gastroenterology* 1991; 26:73–81). In Britain, 10 percent of the population had weekly heartburn with another 21.3 percent experiencing it at least once a month (Thompson, W. G., et al., *Canadian Medical Association Journal* 1982; 126:46–48). Another British study found 31 percent had experienced heartburn at least once in the past six months (Jones, R., et al., *Gut* 1990; 401–405). A review of fifty such studies in developed countries found that the average rate of daily heartburn was 10 percent. As for less developed countries, not many studies exist to document the occurrence levels. However, that does not mean that acid reflux does not exist in those regions; if heartburn did not exist there, there would be no reason for primitive medical treatments such as the aforementioned boiled jasmine root, right?

In a number of studies that looked into age, gender, and racial differences, the disease appears to be more common in adults over the age of fifty than in younger adults. Women, with the exception of those who experience symptoms during pregnancy, appear to be affected later than men. Complications of chronic heartburn tend to affect men more than women. Men tend to account for more cases of esophagitis and men, in general, have a three times greater risk than women of developing esophageal cancer; black men and women have twice as much chance as their white counterparts of developing the deadly complication.

PERSONAL LIVES, PRIVATE PAIN

SO, WHAT DOES this mean to you? Well, it means that you are just the latest in a very long line of individuals who have been diagnosed with this condition.

You join Robin, a fiercely competitive kind of a guy, full of life and great wit. He plays hockey and flies airplanes in his downtime from a hectic job as a business development manager. He is athletic and healthy in every way but one, his reflux.

When Robin was eighteen, he began to experience symptoms of pain and was diagnosed with ulcers. "I was pretty freaked out since I thought ulcers were something for overwrought business people," he said.

It wasn't until he hit his forties that he felt heart palpitations and sought the advice of a physician. The physician ran a number of cardiac tests but finally settled on a diagnosis of GERD.

And Eric is in the group as well. Eric is a lot like Robin, a hard-driving kind of a person in just about every aspect of his life. He is never one to shy away from a challenge, be it putting in extra hours at his job as a business analyst in a high pressure field or going white-water rafting with friends.

In his mid-twenties, Eric found himself having to slow down. He wasn't sleeping well, plagued by a persistent cough and a sore throat. His late-night dinners began to repeat on him, sometimes with painful reminders of the Thai chilis he had consumed earlier. He was diagnosed with GERD shortly thereafter.

Marge, a speech and language pathologist, began having her symptoms while vacationing on the East Coast. After a meal of barbecued ribs, corn on the cob, and beer, she spent the next few days in agonizing pain, vomiting and feeling nauseous. Originally, she thought it was a very bad case of food poisoning but later changed her mind when the symptoms went on for days. She underwent an emergency endoscopic procedure, which revealed scar tissue, a sign of reflux.

She has since undergone many, many other tests that found, among other things, ineffective esophageal motility. Currently, she maintains fairly good health with medication and exercise.

The mini-profiles could go on and on. The point is that this is an illness that, while at times debilitating, has not stood in the way of these people in accomplishing their personal and work-related goals. In addition to these individuals, people such as former U.S. President Bill Clinton, pitcher Jim Palmer, actress Doris Roberts, and singer Lionel Ritchie have all suffered from reflux as well, all while performing their jobs and achieving personal success.

And you will, too. By learning more about the disease and its treatments, you are taking the first step in controlling the disease.

2

〰〰〰

THE DISEASE
AND ITS DIAGNOSIS

At the time of any medical diagnosis, it is not uncommon to feel stunned or sad-
dened or relieved or anything in between. It is also not unusual to be tongue-tied by
the diagnosis, your brain temporarily frozen by emotion, not allowing you to ask questions. You might have been lucky enough to have a doctor who believes in patient
education and who stuffed your hands full of information before departing. Even
then, you likely have a ton of questions about reflux, especially how it happens and
how your doctor knows for sure that this is the answer to your complaints.

When good digestion goes bad

To understand how your doctor arrived at a diagnosis of reflux, it may be helpful
to first understand what happens in a normal digestive process and how it differs from
what is going on in your body. By grasping these differences, you will hopefully see why
you feel what you feel and then understand what is happening to make you feel that
way. Knowing the anatomy of the upper digestive system is important if you are con-
sidering surgery but also in understanding how the medications work. Be prepared,
however, as the following description is rather specific and uses terms that you probably

have not previously heard. Don't feel like you have to absorb it all now. You won't be tested on it. Instead, grasp what you can and use it as a reference in the future. Figure 2 below illustrates the digestive system—though not with quite the detail I provide.

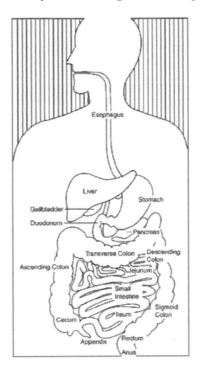

FIGURE 2. THE DIGESTIVE SYSTEM

Source: Courtesy of the National Digestive Disease Information Clearinghouse

The digestive process actually begins in many individuals before food touches the palate as our other senses engage the food that is to be eaten. The sight and smell of food causes acid to be released in the stomach and **mucus** in the form of saliva to be released in the mouth. As the food is broken down into small pieces through chewing, more mucus is released in a digestive process known as **salivation**. The mucus not only provides lubrication to the upper gastrointestinal tract but it also contains an enzyme that begins to break down some of the carbohydrates that are being consumed.

The tongue, a large muscle also blessed with the ability to be a sensory organ, begins another digestive process called **peristalsis**, the movement of substances through the gastrointestinal system through a series of longitudinal and circular muscular contractions. After the food is chewed or as liquid fills the mouth, the tongue propels the substances toward the back of the throat, an area known as the **pharynx**. The upper esophageal sphincter, located approximately behind the knot commonly known as the Adam's apple, opens through an involuntary muscle contraction to allow the food to travel downward.

From there, gravity works with the muscular contractions in the esophagus to push the food down farther. The food passes into the hollow part of the esophagus known as the **lumen**. The lumen is the hollow space throughout the entire gastrointestinal tract, from the esophagus to the anus. The innermost layer of the esophagus, known as the mucosa or tunica mucosa, surrounds the lumen. The layers of the gastrointestinal system are referred to as coats or tunics.

The mucosa is an interesting layer of the intestines as it pretty much lines the entire GI tract, but it acts differently and is formed differently in the various areas. It contains **epithelial cells**, the same category of cells found in several other areas of the body including the skin, the breasts, and the genitals. Here in the esophagus, epithelial cells are arranged in a stratified manner, meaning they are in layers of cells of various sizes and shapes. But in the small intestine, the mucosa is lined with **villi**, little finger-like projections that help to whisk nutrients from the lumen into the bloodstream. In the colon, the job of the mucosa is to reabsorb electrolytes and water from fecal matter. In all places, it acts as a tightly joined immune barrier to the various bacteria and viruses that enter our body through our mouths and aren't killed by the acid and enzymes. In the esophagus, the mucosa is not so much of a stopping point where items are absorbed because food spends little time there; instead, the mucosa acts as a protective barrier.

Beneath the outer most cells in the mucosa is a new layer that has a different function. This layer is known as the **muscularis mucosa**, and it is a thin sheath of muscular cells that stretch just about the length of the esophagus.

The next coat is the **submucosa** or tela submucosa, a layer that is home to esophageal glands that are the source of mucous in the esophagus. The submucosa is also the site of a collection of blood vessels and nerves (**vagus** and sympathetic nerves) that act to connect the mucosa with yet another coat, called the muscularis or tunica muscularis. In this prominent muscular layer, longitudinal muscle fibers (think long, vertical, like the longitudinal lines on a globe) that stretch the length of the esophagus mix with the circular muscle fibers that form rings around the mucosa. The two muscle types work together in a wave-like motion to cause peristalsis. The longitudinal fibers work much like those in a worm: A worm moves by lengthening and shortening itself. The circular muscles in the same layer then contract one after the other, squeezing the food farther through the esophagus. The fibrous or external outer coat acts as a final protective shield for both the esophageal contents and the rest of the body.

The esophagus, as stated before, is about nine inches in length, varying in length proportionally with the height of the individual. It begins at about mid-neck and ends after passing by the trachea, lungs, and heart and through the **diaphragm**, a muscular/membranous structure that divides the **thoracic cavity** (think lungs and heart) from the **abdominal cavity** (liver, kidney, gallbladder, pancreas, spleen, and intestines). The point at which the esophagus breaks through the diaphragm is called the esophageal hiatus. The esophagus joins the stomach a pinch lower at a point called the **cardiac orifice**. It is here that the lower esophageal sphincter is located, opening to allow food into the stomach and closing to keep it there. The time that food or drink take to travel that complex slope is measured in seconds.

The stomach is a very complex organ that changes shape and size depending upon whether it is full or empty, what stage of digestion it is in, or whether the person is lying down or standing up. It can be a thin, hook shape when you are standing and it is empty, or bulbous and distended, say, when you have finished your Thanksgiving dinner and are reclining on the couch in utter exhaustion. The upper part of the stomach is called the **fundus**, the middle part is the **body**, and the lower part is the **antrum** portion. The exit from the stomach is located in the lower part of the stomach and is called the **pylorus**. Depending on the content of the meal, normal digestion can take many minutes or several hours.

The innermost coat or tunic of the stomach is again the mucosa. But here the mucosal cells are arranged in a single layer and are taller and thinner than their counterparts in the esophagus. On closer examination, the mucosal layer reveals an almost honeycomb-like appearance, interspersed with the mouth-like openings of ducts. The ducts travel down toward three different kinds of glands that make secretions of enzymes and mucous. Beneath these cells lies the muscularis mucosa, similar in nature to the same in the esophagus.

One important resident of the mucosa is the **parietal** (literally meaning "wall") **cell,** as this cell is the origin of hydrochloric acid. The cell itself is prompted by one of three sources to create and release the acid. The first source is **acetylcholine**, a neurotransmitter that is released by the vagus nerve in response to the sensations of experiencing the look, the smell, and the taste of food. The chemical is responsible for a number of gastrointestinal motions, but here it activates tiny proton pumps to release the ingredients of the hydrochloric acid. The second source comes from **histamines** that are released when the food causes the stomach to become distended. **G cells,** also in the wall, release **gastrin,** a hormone. The gastrin and the acetylcholine together prompt the release of histamine, a powerful stimulant of gastric secretions. The histamine also activates the proton pump to release the ingredients of hydrochloric acid. Gastrin alone is the third source. It travels through the blood stream to activate the proton pumps into releasing the ingredients of hydrochloric acid. This information will be important to understand when we get to chapter 4 and learn how medical treatments work.

Continuing on with the anatomy of the stomach, the second coat is the submucosa, a tangle of blood vessels, nerves, and connective tissue. The muscular coat lies beneath it and is perhaps one of the most important coats in the series. Three different muscle bands stretch around the stomach lengthwise, circularly, and diagonally, allowing the stomach contents to be squeezed in a variety of combinations of movements. This action helps to obliterate food particles, along with the chemical action provided by the stomach juices. Without the muscles' involuntary action, food would be left to sit in the stomach and slowly digest through the sole action of the gastric juices; one condition that causes this is **gastroparesis**, the paralysis of the stomach muscles that can happen for a variety of reasons but is often associated with diabetes. The final layer is the serous coat or serosa that acts as a barrier between the stomach and the rest of the abdominal cavity.

After the food has been made into a liquid form in the grinding and chemical action of the stomach, it sloshes through the pyloric sphincter into the **duodenum**, the first loop of the intestines, which is about eight inches in length. It is in this loop that the common bile duct opens to dispense bile and pancreatic enzymes, which further act to break down food, which then squeezes through the **jejunum** for the next eight feet before gliding through the **ileum**, the longest of the small intestinal sections at about twelve feet. The layers of the small and large intestine are very much like that of the stomach: the mucosa, which contains epithelial cells and a mucosa muscularis; the submucosa, a mass of nerves and blood vessels; the muscularis, filled with longitudinal and circular muscle fibers; and the serosa, the protective outer coating. All through the small intestine, food is further broken down and nutrients absorbed through a variety of means.

The ileum ends at the **ileocecal valve**, not really a sphincter but a muscular formation nonetheless. The digested matter then enters the **cecum**, a little pocket to which is attached the relatively useless appendix. Here and throughout the **colon**, water and electrolytes are wicked away from the more solid remains of the fecal matter. The fecal matter launches up the **ascending colon**, takes a right at the **hepatic flexure**, travels horizontally through the **transverse colon**, takes another right at the **splenic flexure**, and shoots down the **descending colon,** before snaking through the S-shaped **sigmoid colon**. The waste stores in the expanding **rectum** until it fills, upon which nerves in the rectal wall send a signal that the user has to go to the bathroom. The strong rectal muscles then squeeze the waste through the anal canal and the **anus**. The time food spends in the intestines varies from person to person, meal to meal, from several hours to a few days.

Signs, symptoms, and possible causes

IN A DIGESTIVE process with so many stops and twists and turns, there is much room for dysfunction and disease. Inflammation can occur anywhere along the way, leaving the patient with a condition ending in the suffix "–itis." For example, inflammation of the stomach is gastritis; of the colon, colitis; and of the esophagus, **esophagitis**. Infections caused by bacteria or viruses can lead to ulcerations and inflammation anywhere along the GI tract as well. Diverticula are like little blowouts of the muscular wall, leaving a pouch; this condition can happen anywhere from the esophagus to the rectum but is most common in the colon. Infection in these pouches is called diverticulitis. Beyond the possible inflammation that can occur, the action of the GI tract is dependent upon muscular coordination and thus, motility issues such as irritable bowel syndrome and **dysphasia** (impaired swallowing due at times to uncoordinated muscular response) can happen when involuntary motor responses are not in sync.

In GERD, the acid and pepsin in the stomach do not stay where they are supposed to stay, usually due to a weakened LES (lower esophageal sphincter). The result of this is a backwashing of stomach contents—food, acid, enzymes, mucus, and pepsin—into the esophagus. The esophagus is not designed to handle the acidic refluxate, which can be irritating; at times, this can lead to esophagitis, an inflammation that varies in degree of pain felt from individual to individual. Oftentimes, people complain of heartburn that is worsened after meals, specifically after eating something that is acidic, fatty, alcoholic, or contains items such as chocolate or peppermint; a chart of such foods can be found in chapter 3.

COMMON SIGNS AND SYMPTOMS OF GERD

1. Burning pain in the mid-chest area, often called heartburn
2. Chest pain
3. Sore throat and/or sore mouth
4. Change in voice
5. Vomiting and/or nausea
6. Belching and/or hiccuping
7. Coughing and/or labored breathing
8. Difficulty swallowing and/or the feeling of having food stuck in the throat
9. Interrupted sleep
10. Taste of acid in mouth

In many patients, reflux causes stronger chest pain. This is due to the complex nervous system's wiring of the esophageal/cardiac area of the mid-chest. Because of the anatomical location of the esophagus and the heart, reflux pain that is felt in the area can be confused with cardiac pain and vice versa.

Patrice felt that pain before she was first diagnosed. The mother of two small children, she awoke one night with crushing chest pain. The pain frightened her, especially when it returned not long after that first night. She was certain that an infection in her foot had raced to her heart and was causing her to have heart attack-like symptoms—radiating chest pain, dizziness, and palpitations. She hauled herself to the emergency room, where doctors performed a panel of tests that ruled out a heart condition. They sent Patrice home with a dose of Motrin, telling her anxiety had most likely been the cause of her symptoms. Her primary care physician saw her later when the symptoms returned, and he diagnosed her with reflux.

Vomiting and nausea, symptoms of reflux, generally go hand in hand. This can occur for a number of reasons, not the least of which is that the acid is an irritant in the esophagus, and the esophagus and stomach work to clear it, at times causing vomiting. Other upper gastrointestinal discomfort such as excessive belching and hiccuping can also be signs.

Sierra, a governmental employee, began to shy away from eating out with friends because she would spend the time after the food was consumed hiccuping almost nonstop. "I was just so embarrassed by it," she said. She took this symptom and a persistent sore throat to her gastroenterologist, who diagnosed reflux.

Feeling like food is caught in the throat or experiencing difficulty in swallowing is also a common symptom of reflux. Called dysphagia, it usually starts with food that gets stuck in the esophagus, leaving a feeling of a painful knot at about mid-chest and a sensation of breathlessness. Although it can be muscular in nature, it can also be a sign of long-untreated acid reflux that caused inflammation or scar tissue to narrow the opening of the esophagus, thus forcing stronger contractions to move the food through the smaller opening to the stomach.

Others may experience a continued cough, a reflex to aid the esophagus in clearing the irritant. The burning pain near the breastbone associated with heartburn is related to this occurrence at times. Additionally, some may also experience excessive saliva in the mouth that can be salty or sour in taste; this is often related to the body's attempt to clear the esophagus with the lower-pH saliva.

At times, the acid reflux can propel the stomach acid farther up the esophagus, to the **larynx**, the pharynx, and even the palate; generally, this happens at night when the person is relaxed and sleeping flat in bed, unaware of the occurrence. When this happens repeatedly to the larynx, the person's voice can change, leaving him with a lower, huskier version than he is used to. If the acid and pepsin reach the pharynx time after time, it can cause the person to feel as if he has a sore throat or to have pain upon swallowing. If the acid reaches the palate, it can damage the enamel on the teeth and inflame the oral mucosa, causing a sore mouth. None of these symptoms are particularly uncommon.

Eric, a business analyst, was diagnosed with reflux not long after a friend who is a speech pathologist noticed a change in his voice. For months, he had complained of a sore throat to his doctor who had prescribed an allergy medication to control what was thought to be postnasal drip. Another complaint he had was a constant small cough that kept him up at night. The speech pathologist suggested he see an ear, nose, and throat specialist, who diagnosed the reflux. In controlling the reflux, he was able to eliminate the cough and sore throat, and his voice returned to its normal resonance.

Asthma-like conditions or a worsening of asthma can also be related to reflux. Tightness in the chest, labored breathing, and coughing can occur when the acid is aspirated into the **trachea**, a hollow tube off of the pharynx that leads to the lungs.

Gilda's primary care physician was sure that her difficulty breathing during her regular exercise was a sign of emphysema, related to Gilda's smoking habit she had kicked months before. Nevermind that she had had chest pain and tightness in her chest after drinking coffee or eating spicy foods. The physician said that a test had revealed the beginning stages of the lung disease and that was that. But when the symptoms disappeared after taking an over-the-counter heartburn medication, Gilda began to question the doctor's diagnosis. She saw a gastroenterologist, who ran more tests and found that reflux, not emphysema, was the source of her complaints. She still takes asthma medication to control symptoms as doctors are not completely able to rule out that disease.

COMMON CAUSES

WITH GASTROESOPHAGEAL REFLUX disease, the conditions are usually related to an LES that is weakened intermittently either due to medications or to lifestyle factors. Sometimes, autoimmune diseases, gastrointestinal disorders, or other health conditions such as obesity or pregnancy can also heighten the chances for reflux.

■ ■ ■

COMMON CAUSES OF GERD

1. The presence of hiatal hernia
2. Age
3. Pregnancy
4. Obesity
5. Other diseases
6. Prescription medications
7. Nicotine and alcohol usage

One common cause, especially in people over the age of fifty, is the occurrence of hiatal hernia (see Figure 3), a condition that occurs when a small portion of the stomach slips through the diaphragm into the thoracic cavity. The LES works in conjunction with the opening in the diaphragm; without the pressure from the esophageal hiatus, the LES does not work as well and allows refluxate to travel back into the esophagus. Although not everyone with GERD has a hiatal hernia and conversely not everyone with hiatal hernia has GERD, a strong enough correlation exists that scientists and doctors feel that having a hiatal hernia puts an individual at risk for also having acid reflux.

Whether age itself plays a factor is a matter of debate. However, many prominent physicians in the field of geriatric gastroenterology say that the intestinal muscles, like all muscles in the body, lose tone and experience lessened motility as the body ages. Also, medications that are normally tolerated in younger individuals can have a greater effect on esophageal motility as well as possibly affect the tone of the LES,

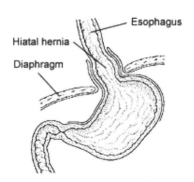

FIGURE 3. HIATAL HERNIA

Source: *Digestive Disease Dictionary,* a publicaiton of the National Institute for Diabetes, Digestive and Kidney Diseases

after all, a muscular valve. This can explain some of the increased rates of GERD in people over the age of fifty. Unfortunately, there is no cure for aging at this time.

Pregnancy by itself is a risk factor for developing reflux. There are a few primary theories as to why this occurs. The first is that the developing fetus causes the relocation of the intestines higher up in the abdominal cavity. The pressure from the increased mass in the digestive organs can force the LES to open and cause the reflux to occur. Also, a fetus' motions inside the uterus can also apply temporary pressure on the stomach. And if you have ever had the bone-jarring experience of having a fetus kick you in the ribs, you can see how this is possible. The second theory is that the different levels of the hormones progesterone and estrogen that are present during pregnancy act to relax the LES pressure. Pregnant women may also crave certain foods or eat at less than optimum times, increasing their chance of developing reflux.

Obesity is seen by some as a risk factor for reflux as well but it is unclear as to exactly why that is. Some theorize that meals consumed by obese individuals are higher in fat and therefore slow stomach emptying, allowing digestion to take longer. Another theory is that bigger meals distend the stomach, putting greater pressure on the LES. Still others suggest that the extra weight around the trunk puts pressure on the stomach, which in turn puts pressure on the LES to open when it shouldn't. But obesity is such a complex topic that such explanations may not be complete or must be used in combination, according to the individual.

Another condition linked to higher rates of reflux is systemic **scleroderma**. This autoimmune disorder causes collagen to be deposited in skin and connective tissues, forming tough patches of skin; in Greek, the name of the disease means "hard skin." In relation to GERD, the majority of the patients with this disease will experience some degree of the scarring of the esophageal muscles, called **fibrosis**. The scar tissue becomes tough and can build up to the point where the lumen is too narrow for food to pass through. A contributing factor can be the use of calcium channel blockers, a category of drugs that can exacerbate GERD but have been shown to help Raynaud's syndrome; that syndrome causes the blood vessels in the hands to constrict, leaves the fingers or fingertips white or blue, and is common in scleroderma patients.

Other gastrointestinal diseases can also cause an increased risk for GERD. For example, Zollinger-Ellison syndrome, a rare disease, can cause increased amounts of gastrin to be produced; as explained above, the gastrin is a prompt for the secretion of hydrochloric acid. Aside from small tumors in the duodenum and the pancreas, the disease is also marked by peptic ulcers that are directly caused by the increased acid. As you can imagine, the increased acid can also reflux up the esophagus.

Delayed gastric emptying, meaning the prolonged period of time that food takes to leave the stomach, can lead to a greater chance of experiencing reflux. The condition is a hallmark of conditions as varied as diabetes mellitus and scleroderma but can also be seen in patients with gastrointestinal diseases characterized by intestinal obstruction through means such as inflammation or scar tissue such as Crohn's disease.

Prescription medications to treat certain conditions can also cause an increase in symptoms in some individuals. In particular, people who take anticholinergic agents, a group of drugs that act to slow the peristaltic waves in the intestines, may find that food sits in their stomach longer, leading to greater degrees of reflux; these agents are often used in people with chronic diarrhea or intestinal spasms due to inflammatory bowel disease or irritable bowel syndrome. Another group of drugs that also act to slow gastrointestinal motility are opiates such as codeine that cause the smooth muscles to slow in their normal responses.

Other drugs that can produce a greater risk of developing reflux symptoms are calcium channel blockers. Used mostly in the treatment of cardiovascular disease such as high blood pressure or coronary artery disease, these drugs open up constricted blood vessels. Another group are tricyclic antidepressants. These drugs work with the neurotransmitters in the brain; unfortunately, many of the same nueruotransmitters work in the gut as well, the medications causing gastrointestinal problems such as constipation and reflux in some patients.

Two nonprescription drugs that are very common in society also have a profound effect on the incidence of reflux: nicotine and alcohol. The evidence from a variety of studies on cigarette smokers and reflux finds that there is an increase in acid reflux among smokers over nonsmokers. But the exact reasons as to why this occurs is not clear. Some scientists feel that it is because smoking causes a decrease in the production of saliva, a valuable resource the body produces that naturally lowers the pH of esophageal acid; with less saliva, the acid can remain in the esophagus and wreck havoc. Other scientists believe that the amount of smoke and toxic gases swallowed during smoking can have an erosive effect on the esophagus and LES. The buildup of the swallowed gases and smoke also can cause greater pressure in the stomach, forcing burping in some. Alcohol, on the other hand, has a direct effect on a) lowering the LES pressure, thus allowing refluxate to travel back up the esophagus and b) delaying gastric emptying since it is known to slow a variety of voluntary and involuntary muscle responses. Additionally, alcohol can make its imbibers sleepy and want to recline after a meal, heightening the chances of reflux.

Outside of the physical conditions and medications linked to higher reflux rates, certain lifestyle factors also play a role in increasing the chances that an individual will experience reflux. Eating high-fat meals, crashing on the couch after a meal, downing caffeine-containing beverages, and bending over not long after eating can bring on the mother of all attacks in people with even the mildest case of reflux. Eating foods that lower the pressure of the LES or increase acid production (peppermint, chocolate, tomato-based foods, onions, garlic, etc.) can also make postmealtime that much more unpleasant.

Taking the Complaint to the Doctor

So, how did your doctor know this was related to reflux and not, say, a heart attack? Or cancer? Or any number of awful diseases that have yet to be discovered? Well, it all begins with the initial exam.

At that first doctor's visit, you likely were weighed and had your blood pressure and temperature taken. A nurse or medical assistant may have asked how tall you were and why you were there that day. Then, the doctor likely assessed your health in the past and in the present, making sure to ask about any health problems that run in the family. Likely, you were asked about whether you smoked and drank and, if so, how often and how much. This is called a medical history and it is pretty standard stuff.

Then, the doctor likely examined you further, poking and prodding your body in a variety of spots while assessing your reaction. Because this part of the exam greatly relies on your input, it is really important to not hold back here. Don't think that you are being a big baby if you complain about waking up every night with a scorching pain in your chest. Your doctor needs to know this information and whatever else you've got to properly evaluate the situation.

After assessing your physical symptoms and history, he or she will decide exactly which tests are needed to further diagnose the condition and when they should be scheduled. Obviously, if you are bent over, clutching your chest, and more nauseous than you have ever felt, your doctor may decide that you need to be in the emergency room immediately, having all kinds of cardiac tests as well as GI tests. But if you simply describe the taste of acid in your mouth, he or she may tell you to chew on a few pills and ask you to hang out in the waiting room to see what happens.

Unfortunately, there isn't one blood or breath test that absolutely signals without error that reflux is what you have. Therefore, your doctor likely ordered at least one test, if not a few. These tests include endoscopic procedures, barium Xrays, esophageal manometry, 24-hour ambulatory pH tests, and the Bernstein test as well as other tests to rule out other conditions.

Esophageogastroduodenoscopy (EGD)

Endoscopic procedures can be called by a number of different names, all highlighting the area that is to be examined. For example, a colonoscopy examines the length of the colon while a sigmoidoscopy only makes it up to the sigmoid. Similarly the esophagoscopy won't go nearly as far as the gastroscopy or the **esophageogastroduodenoscopy (EGD).** But what is common with all of the tests is the tool with which they are performed, the endoscope. This is a long, thin, usually black, snakelike tool that is outfitted with a lenspiece and controls on the external end and a fiberoptic camera, cool lighting, and biopsy snare or dilation equipment on the part that is placed in the patient.

For the upper gastrointestinal endoscopic procedures, the test begins with the patient not eating or drinking for eight hours prior to the test time. This allows the stomach to empty. For this reason, it is fairly easy to schedule this test first thing in the morning. The patient is sedated through an intravenous line, usually with a mix of the painkiller Demerol and the sedative Valium, as well as a short-term amnesia drug called Versed; sometimes, a short-term anesthesia is used in place of these medications. The patient lies flat on his or her back as the physician first inserts a bite plane to protect the equipment and the patient's teeth. Some doctors also spray the back of the throat with a numbing medication to alleviate the feeling of choking as the scope is inserted into the mouth and down the esophagus.

Using the light and camera to see the esophagus, the doctor is able to assess any changes in the mucosa. He or she can also take biopsies of the mucosa here as well as in the stomach and duodenum. The biopsies, generally painless in nature, are sent to a pathologist to determine any changes in normal cell patterns. The patient is sent to recovery following the procedure.

Because of the sedation and the lingering effects of the Versed, the majority of hospitals require that a patient undergoing the procedure have a friend or relative not only escort the patient but also hear the results of the test. Additionally, it is a good idea for him or her to take the rest of the day off of work, school, or household responsibilities as the patient will likely be groggy.

While the test is fairly easy on the patient if he or she is properly sedated, the drawback for the doctors is that it doesn't allow for them to see if there are any problems with swallowing and also may not pick up a case of GERD that is characterized by no changes in the esophageal mucosa. The upside is that it allows the doctor not only to see the esophagus, stomach, and duodenum but also to take samples for study.

Barium Xray

Barium Xray studies also require the same prep, by and large. Again, there are a variety of studies using barium, a white rock that is pulverized and suspended in liquid, as a contrast. But for the purposes of diagnosing GERD, you will likely not have it inserted into your anus. Instead, the test is referred to as the upper GI or the barium swallow.

For the test, some patients whose doctors are also using air as a second contrast will be given a fizzy drink to swallow quickly before they have to chug down a heavy cup of barium. Usually, this is accompanied by a strong urge to burp. Don't. For those whose doctors are not using the double contrast, straight barium is consumed. The key to getting through the taste of the chalky material is to a) be sure to continue to breathe as not doing so simply heightens the gag reflex and b) drink as fast as you can. Some people simply cannot choke the barium down and must have a thin, flexible tube inserted up the nose and down the throat to pump the barium in. If this is the case, the tube is generally withdrawn quickly and painlessly after the procedure is done.

The Xray pictures are taken at specific intervals to determine whether or not there is normal motility in the patient. The patient may also be required to roll around several times or be gently shaken to coat the stomach with the barium. The test will pick up any abnormal structures in the esophagus and stomach such as a narrowing in the esophagus or a hiatal hernia. However, it won't be able to detail any changes in the mucosa. For this reason, it is often necessary to do this test in conjunction with others.

After the procedure is done, the patient is allowed to go home. Over the next day or so, the barium will begin to pass through the intestines. As it does, it will become more congealed. For this reason, some doctors prescribe a laxative such as Milk of Magnesia to help the patient pass the barium.

Esophageal manometry

The **esophageal manometry** test is not a very pleasant test to undergo but may be necessary if the patient experiences pain or difficulty in swallowing. If the patient is a candidate for surgical intervention, the test may be required prior to surgery to rule out any motility disorders.

The prep for the test begins about a week before the scheduled date. At that point, patients are asked to refrain from taking any proton pump inhibitors. A few days before the test, all histamine H_2 blockers are stopped. Antacids, the final recourse for relief, are generally prohibited a day or two before the test. On the day of the test, the patient must refrain from eating about six hours before the allotted time to prevent any vomiting of stomach contents during the test.

Before the test begins, the patient's nose and back of the throat may be sprayed with a local anesthetic to ease the passing of a tube outfitted with small sensors through the nose, down the esophagus, and into the stomach. The process is uncomfortable but blessedly brief; probably the worst part of it is that the motion of the tube down the throat causes a strong gag reflex, often followed by retching. For the next forty-five minutes to about two hours, the patient must remain still and refrain from swallowing unless directed to do so by the technician. This is a difficult task at best since the tube can be an irritant in the throat. It helps to focus on an object or on breathing patterns to take your mind off the discomfort and try to relax. The better able you are to relax and follow the technician's orders, the faster the test will go and the less time you will spend undergoing its torture.

The technician will use the tube and its sensors to test the strength of esophageal muscles and their coordination during the swallowing process. The tube and sensors are slowly withdrawn, stopping at specific spots along the esophagus to obtain a better picture of the whole process. After the results are gathered and interpreted, the doctor receives a copy he or she can share with the patient.

24-hour ambulatory pH monitoring

In some cases, the esophageal manometry concludes with the withdrawing of the instrument only to have yet another instrument placed in a similar manner. Thankfully, the equipment used for the **24-hour ambulatory pH monitoring** test is thinner and much easier to tolerate.

This test is used as a way to prove reflux if physical evidence such as esophagitis is not proven through other tests such as endoscopy or barium Xray or if the patient has some of the extraesophageal manifestations of reflux such as asthma or a persistent cough. Sometimes, it is used in people who are having poor treatment results and who did not have esophagitis on examination. Commonly, it is used preoperatively to confirm a case of reflux. Additionally, it is used following surgery if a patient continues to experience reflux symptoms despite the surgical intervention.

In this test, the instrument is inserted, with the outer portion taped into place on the face and attached to a small, battery-powered recording device, and worn for one full day. The device is able to measure the fluctuations in esophageal acidity while you eat, sleep, work, and play. In a person with a normal digestive response, the pH in the esophagus is at a healthy level if it is at a pH of four or above for the vast majority of the day, perhaps slipping below four a small fraction of the recorded time; in people with reflux, the test will show greater and more frequent dips in the pH, especially following a meal or while reclining.

While the test is in progress, the patient is encouraged to live as he or she normally would without reflux. For example, the patient is told not to avoid the foods he or she would usually nix or to have that scotch before bedtime, if that is usual. Without the protection of the medications, the patient will certainly feel all the symptoms and then some, all of which are recorded on the device. Some devices carry the option of pressing certain buttons when certain sensations occur such as severe chest pain or when the patient partakes in some activity, such as when retiring for the night. At the end of the test, the monitor is swiftly removed through the nose and the data is downloaded for analysis.

Some might be relieved to know that new equipment is being developed to reduce the worst part of the test, the feeling of having the cord up the nose and down the throat for an entire day. Scientists are developing a monitor that can be secured in the throat with dissolvable stitches. The device then sends a signal to an external monitor for the time needed. After the test concludes, the monitor's stitches dissolve and the monitor, no bigger than a pill, is excreted from the body through the normal waste process.

Other tests

There are other tests that doctors use for diagnosing other possible causes of reflux. One of the older and not very often used tests to determine whether a patient has reflux is the **Bernstein test**. Based on the theory that the hydrochloric acid from the stomach causes pain associated with reflux, the test involves the dripping of a man-made solution of hydrochloric acid as well as saline or salt water down the throat of the patient, alternating one with the other and then combining both. The fluids travel through a nasogastric tube placed about two-thirds of the way down the esophagus. Just as with the other tests, the prep for this one involves the absence of food for six to eight hours.

If the patient experiences pain with the acid that is relieved with the following course of saline, it tells the doctor that the esophagus is sensitive to the acid. If pain occurs with the saline or with a combination of the two, it can indicate that there is a problem with swallowing. Obviously, the scope of the test is limited as it can only diagnose those with classic heartburn-like symptoms. For those with a persistent cough or other extraesophageal symptoms, the test will likely find nothing. Because of this, few people are subjected to the test.

Another test measures the stomach's capacity for emptying. Called **scintigraphy**, the test involves consuming a food, such as cornflakes or scrambled eggs, that has been laced with a radionuclide. The radionuclide will glow in a photograph made by a gamma camera but otherwise has no taste and leaves the body fairly quickly. This test is important for people in whom stomach emptying may be delayed due to gastroparesis or obstruction due to inflammation or scar tissue.

Another optional test that uses a piece of technology called the **spectrophotometer** helps to measure the presence of bilirubin, a liver by-product. In these patients, the damage is done by the bile that travels from the gallbladder down the common bile duct and into the duodenum; instead of going farther down the small intestine, in some individuals the bile travels backwards through the stomach and up into the esophagus. The bile, in which bilirubin is a plentiful ingredient, then causes the pain in the esophagus. The equipment here is the same as the pH monitoring equipment except that it is sensitive to the greater pH of the bilirubin. Oftentimes, an individual who is undergoing pH monitoring will also undergo monitoring for bilirubin.

Finally, some doctors prescribe reflux medication for a patient without testing for the condition. The theory here is that the patient who responds to the medication has reflux.

ARRIVING AT THE DIAGNOSIS

WITH ALL THAT could be going on, how did your doctor arrive at reflux as the end diagnosis? Usually, he or she does so through a process of elimination. With chest pain, for example, it might be a heart attack or it might be an attack more closely related to that fatty meal you consumed about fifteen minutes before bedtime. If you have a problem breathing, the cigarette smoke you've been inhaling might be causing lung damage, or it might be weakening the LES, causing reflux. With a pile of tests and results and their correlation with the symptoms, a doctor can usually rule out one or more conditions and settle on a diagnosis of reflux. Here are some of the conditions often ruled out:

- *Cardiac conditions* can be often confused with reflux. However, a battery of cardiac examinations including a stress test, an electrocardiogram (involving the attachment of electrodes to the body to record cardiac activity), and a cardiac enzyme test (involving the measuring of specific enzymes in the blood that are released during a heart attack), among others, can determine if a heart attack has occurred or is occurring. This is not to say that a person experiencing a heart attack won't also have reflux but it can determine recent chest pain as noncardiac chest pain or NCCP, a common reflux sign.
- There is no specific test to rule out a case of **costochondritis**, the inflammation of the joints that connect the sternum to the ribs. There is also no set cause for the painful condition. However, cases of costochondritis generally last for a few days and are adequately treated with the application of heat and cold in intervals and with the use of pain relievers.
- **Achalasia** is a rare disorder in the esophagus that is caused by a lack of nerve response. People with this condition lack the proper response to food in the esophagus, leaving the LES closed. The retention of the food in the intestines causes the esophagus to distend and can lead to chest pain that is similar to that which is felt by a GERD patient. To rule this condition out, doctors rely on the readings of the esophageal manometry.
- Asthma can be a very serious lung condition caused by the constriction of the bronchial tubes and marked by wheezing, difficulty in breathing, and coughing. Some people with reflux share those symptoms after they breathe in the refluxate and others have both conditions, making a sure diagnosis difficult. To diagnose asthma, doctors can order a number of pulmonary function tests and Xrays. After a diagnosis of either GERD or asthma is made and the patient doesn't respond to treatment, often the other condition is suspected either as the culprit or as a co-conspirator.
- **Helicobacter pylori** is the name of tiny bacteria that can cause a lot of problems as it is the chief culprit of ulceration in the stomach and duodenum. There are a few different ways to find out if the bacteria is the cause for the ulcerations, including a blood test or a stool test, but a common way of doing so is a breath test that measures levels of carbon dioxide emitted by the bacteria. Also,

a biopsy of the affected gastric mucosa will show whether or not the bacteria are present. The interesting thing about the bacteria is that they act to suppress gastric acid secretion in some people. While that might seem like a good thing for patients with GERD, the bacteria, though not always causing symptoms, has also been linked with the formation of certain stomach cancers so doctors find it important to eradicate the bacteria when it is found. The flip side to that is that the acid secretion usually increases after the bacteria is gone, leading to the symptoms of GERD in some. So treatment for the bacteria often includes acid-suppressing medication as well as antibiotics to kill off the bacteria.

■ Zollinger-Ellison syndrome is very rare and occurs mainly in people between the ages of thirty and sixty. It shares some of the same symptoms of GERD but is characterized by the overproduction of acid due to gastrin-producing tumors in the duodenum and pancreas. A blood test to measure levels of gastrin in the blood as well as biopsies of the tumors can help to ascertain this diagnosis.

SO NOW WHAT?

NOW, IT IS your decision about what will happen. Clearly, you can follow the doctor's orders, take medication, or, failing that option, have surgery and see what happens. Or you can try supplementing that with some alternative medicine or lifestyle modifications as well. Or you can do nothing.

In this book, specific chapters have been devoted to options in lifestyle modification, medication, alternative medication, and surgery. However, there is always the option of going it alone, either with or without over-the-counter aids. It may be that you have a mild, transient case of reflux that you feel you can control, or it may be that you find it easier to pop a few antacids during your daily attacks than go through the rigmarole of the testing and hassle of taking daily medication.

Whatever the case, having reflux that is not contained through lifestyle modification and going without treatment in the long term may lead to drastic consequences. You should know this if you plan on embarking on this course at any time just as anyone who is embarking on a medical or surgical treatment plan should also be appraised of the risks.

To start, prolonged inflammation and healing of the mucosa in cases where esophagitis exists causes the buildup of scar tissue in the esophagus, effectively narrowing the lumen. This scar tissue can inhibit swallowing, the esophagus becoming so narrow at times that only liquids can pass through. Strictures can be treated through the endoscopic procedure known as dilation but this is a painful process that must be repeated regularly.

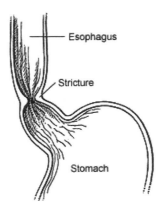

FIGURE 4. STRICTURE

Source: *Digestive Disease Dictionary,* a publicaiton of the National Institute for Diabetes, Digestive and Kidney Diseases

Barrett's esophagus is a precancerous condition of the esophagus that occurs in people who have long-standing GERD. It is caused by the erosive action of the refluxed acid on the sensitive mucosa. In time, the mucosal cells can alter their arrangement from stratified to columnar, a change that is known as **dysplasia**. In all intestinal cancers, the development of dysplasia brings with it the *possibility* of cancer, meaning that not all people who have dysplasia will develop cancer, but some of those who develop cancer first were found to have dysplasia. The rate of Barrett's esophagus patients who develop cancer is about one percent per year. As the American Cancer Society explains it, that means out of one hundred people with Barrett's esophagus, one will develop cancer in one year.

The condition usually is not considered reversible. However, some advances have been made to try to contain the condition, if not reverse it. One, called photodynamic therapy (PDT), involves the use of a light-sensitive drug that reacts to a laser's light to slough off the damaged mucosa, allowing for healthier mucosa to rebuild itself. Another, called endoscopic mucosal resection (EMR), allows for the removal of large sections of precancerous and stage 1 cancerous sections of affected mucosa to be removed without affecting the structure of the esophagus. Controversy over the beneficial effects of the techniques continues, and there are no long-term results available for them. Short of using these procedures, doctors who care for patients with Barrett's esophagus generally try to keep the reflux in check while performing regular endoscopic exams and taking biopsies to check the condition's progress.

Esophageal cancer is ultimately the worst outcome of untreated reflux. It can develop with or without a previous diagnosis of Barrett's esophagus, although people with Barrett's have a fifty times greater risk of developing esophageal cancer than those without it. Esophageal cancer treatment varies with the stage in which it is detected; those in the earlier stages have the best chance for long-term survival. However, it bears repeating here that thirteen thousand Americans die of the disease each year.

3

※

LIFESTYLE CHANGES

Things we do in our everyday lives—whether actively or passively—make a significant impact on our health. If you live in an area with a lot of smog, you have a higher chance of developing respiratory illness. If you eat a high-fat diet, you run the risk of developing a number of cancers. If you keep your weight within a reasonable range, you reduce the possibility of becoming ill from a number of diseases.

With GERD, lifestyle factors can also have a giant impact. For example, if you smoke, drink alcohol, and eat a high-fat meal, you run a greater risk of having a reflux episode than if you abstain from the alcohol and tobacco and eat more sensibly. In fact, nearly every aspect of our lives—from the way we dress to the way we sleep, from the way we eat to when we eat—may have some impact on the severity and frequency of reflux attacks.

By making certain lifestyle modifications, we exercise some measure of control over these episodes. And not all of the changes are as huge as stopping smoking, breaking a habit that has often been compared with eliminating a heroin addiction. Some are simple: wear looser clothing, prop up the torso when sleeping, and eat smaller meals. Yet the payoff for such simple alterations can be a measurable increase in comfort.

STOPPING SMOKING

EVEN WITHOUT REFLUX, there are plenty of reasons to quit smoking. Smoking causes a number of obvious cancers—including lung, oral, pharyngeal, laryngeal, and esophageal—and is suspected to be a significant factor in a number of other cancers such as colon cancer and bladder cancer. That doesn't even touch on the financial issue of smoking, including the basic cost of the habit (cigarettes run over $12 a pack in some places in the country, clothing is ruined by burns and intractable smell, smoking-related diseases stand to cost the individuals thousands of dollars, etc.) and the growing social stigma attached to the habit.

But when a person with GERD smokes, there appears to be a direct impact on the condition. In numerous studies, smokers were monitored during various tests such as esophageal manometry and the 24-hour ambulatory pH test as well as with experiments measuring LES pressure as they smoked. The various experiments concluded that while the test participants smoked and for a few minutes afterward, the LES relaxed, allowing acid to splash into the esophagus. Still more studies note that those who smoke and have erosive esophagitis have longer healing times, likely due to the continued irritating effects of smoke on the epithelium. To be perfectly fair, there have also been a smaller number of studies that do not find LES relaxation during smoking. But the point is that smoking is not a good way to improve one's health and it may have a very real impact on reflux.

> ### FINDING HELP WITH SMOKING CESSATION
>
>
>
> QUITTING SMOKING is a difficult but worthwhile proposition for most. And it has probably never been easier. Perhaps the best way to quit for you is to gain the support of loved ones, to consult a trusted primary care physician, and to discuss all of the options to find the best and most economical way to do so.
>
> In the past two decades, an arsenal of products have been developed to help a smoker quit; think nicotine patches, the prescription drug Zyban, nicotine gum, inhalers, nasal sprays, and behavioral alteration programs and you are thinking of some of the latest smoking cessation programs to debut. The options range in price from free to a few hundred dollars and report varying success rates.
>
> *continued*

Organized programs have also helped thousands to quit. For more information, call the American Lung Association at 1-800-LUNG-USA, visit them online at *www.lungusa.org* or check out their on-line smoking cessation site at *www.ffsonline.org*. Other web sites that support smoking cessation include *www.quitnet.com*, a Boston University program that offers a fee-based as well as a free on-line program, and *www.nicotine-anonymous.org*, a program based on the twelve-step approach to breaking addictions that sponsors meetings in every state and many countries.

REDUCING OR ELIMINATING ALCOHOL

ALCOHOL IS WIDELY used in modern culture, and its presence is seen pervasively in the media. Companies that make alcoholic beverages splash their names on race cars, build stadiums, fund universities, and sponsor some of the swankiest fundraisers. Ads for certain alcoholic beverages have been raised to an art form in that copies of the ads are collected, while different manufacturers' ads are nearly omnipresent and feature thin, glamorous models and shapely bottles.

But if the reality of alcohol use was truly shown in ads, it would paint a far different picture. In the extreme, alcohol, as a drug, can have a damaging effect on individuals, families, and societies if it is abused; it can lead to brain damage, liver damage, and a host of other serious illnesses, leading to death in some. Even in moderate use, its empty calories can cause weight gain and its inebriating effects can cause some to lose inhibition, consuming more than they normally would. Further, alcohol can have a caustic effect on the inflamed mucosa of erosive esophagitis, causing a burning pain as it is swallowed. While moderate use of alcohol may give some who have GERD pause, it should also be considered that alcohol has been shown to lower the LES pressure and delay gastric emptying, leading to nasty bouts of reflux in some.

For some people with GERD, having one occasional drink with a meal may have no discernable effect. However, others immediately feel the effects and must be assiduous in their avoidance of alcohol.

For the occasional drinker, there are plenty of other alternatives to alcohol including herbal, noncaffeinated iced tea, plain and flavored water, and certain fruit juices; if you feel the urge to imbibe, choose a drink that does not use certain fruit juices (tomato, grapefruit, orange juices, or sour mixes come to mind), caffeine (colas or coffee), or carbonated items (other sodas) as these mixers can intensify a reflux reaction; also, some avoid naturally carbonated beverages such as beer as they can lead to belching, an inducement to reflux. You may also try watering the alcohol down to reduce the amount that is consumed. And be sure to avoid lying down after drinking alcohol (see below).

FINDING HELP WITH QUITTING DRINKING

IF YOU feel you might have an addictive issue with alcohol, you may want to first consult your doctor and then seek treatment. You may be referred to a residential treatment program, a psychotherapist who treats addiction issues, or a support group, depending on the severity of the issue and your means. One sound jumping off point for seeking treatment for many is to join Alcoholics Anonymous (*www.alcoholics-anonymous.org*). This organization has helped millions to stop drinking and stay sober. The web site carries information about all of its American and international groups, some of which have twenty-four-hour hotlines.

LOSING WEIGHT

JIM IS ONE of those guys who loves to eat. When reflux first entered his life, he took medication to control the symptoms so he could continue to indulge . . . so much so that he packed 250 pounds onto his five-foot nine-inch frame. However, reflux soon hit again, despite medication. Through a modified, albeit bland, diet, he was able to reduce his weight to 168 pounds in one year, further reducing his reflux symptoms. Annabel, the chef who created the recipes in the second half of the book, was much the same. When she was at her heaviest, she found herself having to sit up in order to sleep, leaving gravity to help ease the burning pain in her esophagus. After losing twenty-five pounds, she found that she also lost the majority of the signs and symptoms of her reflux. Jim and Annabel have discovered what is suspected as a prompt for reflux symptoms: being overweight or obese.

Individuals who are overweight or obese already face a serious health risk, as being heavier has been linked to increased rates of high blood pressure, cardiovascular disease, diabetes mellitus, and certain cancers. With GERD, being overweight or obese

Body Mass Index Table

	Normal						Overweight					Obese										Extreme Obesity														
BMI	19	20	21	22	23	24	25	26	27	28	29	30	31	32	33	34	35	36	37	38	39	40	41	42	43	44	45	46	47	48	49	50	51	52	53	54
Height (inches)												Body Weight (pounds)																								
58	91	96	100	105	110	115	119	124	129	134	138	143	148	153	158	162	167	172	177	181	186	191	196	201	205	210	215	220	224	229	234	239	244	248	253	258
59	94	99	104	109	114	119	124	128	133	138	143	148	153	158	163	168	173	178	183	188	193	198	203	208	212	217	222	227	232	237	242	247	252	257	262	267
60	97	102	107	112	118	123	128	133	138	143	148	153	158	163	168	174	179	184	189	194	199	204	209	215	220	225	230	235	240	245	250	255	261	266	271	276
61	100	106	111	116	122	127	132	137	143	148	153	158	164	169	174	180	185	190	195	201	206	211	217	222	227	232	238	243	248	254	259	264	269	275	280	285
62	104	109	115	120	126	131	136	142	147	153	158	164	169	175	180	186	191	196	202	207	213	218	224	229	235	240	246	251	256	262	267	273	278	284	289	295
63	107	113	118	124	130	135	141	146	152	158	163	169	175	180	186	191	197	203	208	214	220	225	231	237	242	248	254	259	265	270	278	282	287	293	299	304
64	110	116	122	128	134	140	145	151	157	163	169	174	180	186	192	197	204	209	215	221	227	232	238	244	250	256	262	267	273	279	285	291	296	302	308	314
65	114	120	126	132	138	144	150	156	162	168	174	180	186	192	198	204	210	216	222	228	234	240	246	252	258	264	270	276	282	288	294	300	306	312	318	324
66	118	124	130	136	142	148	155	161	167	173	179	186	192	198	204	210	216	223	229	235	241	247	253	260	266	272	278	284	291	297	303	309	315	322	328	334
67	121	127	134	140	146	153	159	166	172	178	185	191	198	204	211	217	223	230	236	242	249	255	261	268	274	280	287	293	299	306	312	319	325	331	338	344
68	125	131	138	144	151	158	164	171	177	184	190	197	203	210	216	223	230	236	243	249	256	262	269	276	282	289	295	302	308	315	322	328	335	341	348	354
69	128	135	142	149	155	162	169	176	182	189	196	203	209	216	223	230	236	243	250	257	263	270	277	284	291	297	304	311	318	324	331	338	345	351	358	365
70	132	139	146	153	160	167	174	181	188	195	202	209	216	222	229	236	243	250	257	264	271	278	285	292	299	306	313	320	327	334	341	348	355	362	369	376
71	136	143	150	157	165	172	179	186	193	200	208	215	222	229	236	243	250	257	265	272	279	286	293	301	308	315	322	329	338	343	351	358	365	372	379	386
72	140	147	154	162	169	177	184	191	199	206	213	221	228	235	242	250	258	265	272	279	287	294	302	309	316	324	331	338	346	353	361	368	375	383	390	397
73	144	151	159	166	174	182	189	197	204	212	219	227	235	242	250	257	265	272	280	288	295	302	310	318	325	333	340	348	355	363	371	378	386	393	401	408
74	148	155	163	171	179	186	194	202	210	218	225	233	241	249	256	264	272	280	287	295	303	311	319	326	334	342	350	358	365	373	381	389	396	404	412	420
75	152	160	168	176	184	192	200	208	216	224	232	240	248	256	264	272	279	287	295	303	311	319	327	335	343	351	359	367	375	383	391	399	407	415	423	431
76	156	164	172	180	189	197	205	213	221	230	238	246	254	263	271	279	287	295	304	312	320	328	336	344	353	361	369	377	385	394	402	410	418	426	435	443

FIGURE 5. ARE YOU A HEALTHY WEIGHT?

Source: Adapted from *Clinical Guidelines on the Identification, Evaluation, and Treatment of Overweight and Obesity in Adults: The Evidence Report*

may mean more episodes. No one is exactly sure why this is so, but a number of valid theories abound. For one, carrying extra weight in the abdominal region can cause greater pressure in the belly, forcing the stomach upwards and putting pressure on the LES. Another theory is that overweight and obese people tend to eat larger and fattier meals than their thinner counterparts, a habit that also places pressure on the stomach. In treating reflux with surgery, being overweight or obese can add to the risk for complications during and after the surgery and in general require more skill of the surgeon.

Determining whether you are a healthy weight or not depends upon your height and your weight. The National Institutes of Health suggests multiplying your weight (in pounds) by 704.5, then dividing that result by your height (in inches) once, and then again. You will come up with a number that generally runs below 40. If that number is between 18.5 and 25, your weight is considered to be healthy. If that number is 25.1 to 30, you are considered overweight. If that number is greater than 30, you are obese. See Figure 5 to help determine your ideal weight.

FINDING HELP WITH LOSING WEIGHT

WHATEVER THE reason, a person who is overweight or obese and has reflux may reduce symptoms simply by losing a portion of his or her weight. There are a number of ways to accomplish this, all of which require effort from patient, encouragement from the patient's loved ones, and supervision from the physician.

Diets are perhaps the most non-invasive way to lose weight but are by no means a quick fix, as a majority of the most successful dieters slowly shed weight, losing on average less than two pounds per week. Reflux may complicate matters, as finding the right diet to accomplish the goal of long-standing weight loss while avoiding symptoms can be a difficult proposition. Many doctors will recommend tried and true yet low cost or free programs such as Weight Watchers (*www.weightwatchers.com*) or a twelve-step program such as Overeaters Anonymous (www.overeatersanonymous.org), while superimposing further dietary restrictions such as avoiding many of the reflux triggers listed later in the chapter.

When diets alone are not helpful in achieving weight loss, the physician may take the next step and prescribe certain weight-loss medications such

continued

as Meridia (sibutramine), a drug that acts on appetite control centers in the brain, or Xenical (orlistat), a drug that acts to bond with enzymes that break down fat and allow the fat to travel through the intestines undigested, along with the diet (other weight-loss medications are being developed and will likely debut in the next few years).

If these weight loss methods fail or if the person's obesity is causing other potentially deadly conditions, a doctor may refer the patient to a surgeon. In obese or overweight patients, some surgeons may suggest combining the laparoscopic Nissen fundoplication to tighten the LES with a weight-loss surgery such as silicone-adjusted gastric banding or a Roux-en Y gastric bypass. Both weight-loss surgeries have been shown in studies to ease reflux symptoms while allowing pounds to be shed.

EXERCISING . . . BUT NOT TOO VIGOROUSLY

EXERCISE REDUCES WEIGHT. Exercise reduces stress. Exercise improves digestion. Exercise lubricates the joints. Exercise improves immune function. Exercise sharpens the mind. Exercise strengthens cardiovascular output. We could go on in this stream of thinking forever about the benefits of exercise, but let's just focus on the top three here in relation to the way that these benefits pertain to GERD.

Exercise reduces weight in most people. And we aren't talking about training for a marathon or going mountain climbing. For a 155-pound adult, simply walking for an hour at a moderate pace burns 246 calories, while raking leaves burns 281 in the same amount of time, and jogging at a rate of 12 minutes per mile can burn 563 calories in 60 minutes. Because the National Institutes of Health say that more than half of all adult Americans are either overweight or obese, most of us could stand to do a little more than we are already doing. And since carrying extra weight around may be a factor in GERD symptoms, it might be more than worthwhile to do even a little more than that.

Exercise reduces stress in most people. Physically, it allows you to sweat out your anxieties and put your worries at least temporarily out of your mind as you focus on the task at hand. Exercise can help you accomplish goals, such as weight loss or training for an event, which in turn can reward you with higher self-esteem. Also, at some level of exercise, endorphins, naturally occurring opiates, are released in the brain and can help to control pain responses in the body and reduce the feeling of tension. It is interesting to note that endorphins are also released during sex as well as while deeply relaxed or while laughing.

Exercise improves digestion in most people. Despite what your mother told you about jumping in the water after a full meal ("You're gonna get a cramp!"), mild to moderate exercise after a meal can actually help to improve digestion. To walk around the block, to clear the table and do the dishes, to take in a postbreakfast tai chi class improves the motility of the stomach and the intestines, especially helpful in those with sluggish digestion.

Not all exercise is the same, however; some forms of exercise can actually exacerbate the condition. Jumping up and down during high-impact aerobics, lifting heavy weights as well as vigorously biking, jogging, hiking, or running can cause strain or movement enough to force the stomach contents to splash into the esophagus. Doing crunches or sit-ups or simply bending at the waist can also force a surge of acid to the palate.

John can testify to that. He feels that his hiatal hernia was likely caused by physically overexerting himself while weight lifting. "There is a small group of GERDies, myself included, who, before they had their GERD, ate nutritiously, exercised regularly, were already trim at the waist, and nonsmokers, that find themselves with GERD after a consistent habit of improper lifting or even one, single traumatic lift," he said.

FINDING HELP TO START EXERCISING

STARTING EXERCISING is never easy, especially if you haven't done it in awhile. But that doesn't mean it can't be done. The first step in getting moving is to consult your doctor to make sure it is safe to do so. He or she may also be helpful in suggesting the type and frequency of activity to which you would be best suited.

Many people with GERD find that they are more inclined to participate in gentle exercises and movements such as bending at the knee, walking at a moderate pace, practicing tai chi, or performing certain yoga positions, these movements can be easy enough to allow for extra movement without the increase in reflux. Many of these classes are offered at economical rates at your local YMCA (see *www.YMCA.net* to find one near you) or Jewish community center (most open to the public, see *www.jcca.org* for a location near you).

continued

To take the financial stress out of working out at a gym or in a class, be sure to try the exercises first. Some gyms offer free but brief memberships or passes to classes to allow people to test drive the programs. Video-tapes of tai chi or yoga, for example, can usually be borrowed from the local library or rented from a well-stocked video store first to allow a trial run before investing in a class.

DRESSING SENSIBLY

THE STOMACH, IN some ways, is like a balloon, the contents of which, after a meal, is food. Common sense dictates that if you put extra pressure on the abdomen, then the stomach just might react by pressuring the LES to open up and forcing the contents to splash up into the esophagus or farther.

But many people don't see this in terms of what they wear. At Thanksgiving, for example, they may don a strangling pair of control-top pantyhose or a pair of slacks that are cinched tightly by a belt, knowing full well that they intend to eat more during this one meal than many residents of poor countries will eat in a month. Others might purchase a stiff pair of form-fitting jeans without sitting down in them while still in the dressing room, thereby not realizing just how painful that can be. Or some insist that they still fit into a size ten when a size fourteen might actually make them appear more like a human and less like a giant stuffed sausage.

Sue Ann altered her clothing after learning that it could ease her pain. "After I was diagnosed, I switched to elastic waistbands and loose clothing," she said. "I was too ignorant prediagnosis to know that this would help."

TIPS FOR A MORE COMFORTABLE FIT

TO REDUCE the amount of constriction that clothing can place on the mid-section, there are a few things that people can do, outside of purchasing that roomier size. For both men and women, there are many styles in slacks,

continued

jeans, or skirts that offer forgiving, belt-free waistlines—some made with gentle, hidden stretches of elastic—without sacrificing style. If you can't get away with that daily in the business setting, try unbuttoning at the waist and wearing a shirt or blouse over the undone closure. As soon as you are able to slip into something less restrictive, ditch the binding clothing in favor of drawstring or elasticized waists. For women, a dress without a defined waist can be a godsend; also, pregnancy pantyhose offer all of the elegance of the control-top variety with a more comfortable fit.

SLEEPING ON AN ANGLE

GRAVITY, AS IT is known, is what holds things on the Earth and keeps the Earth spinning around the sun. In people with reflux, gravity can help to keep what has been produced or consumed in the stomach and not in the esophagus, or it can work against the patient by allowing just the opposite to occur.

Of course, all of this depends upon the angle in which the individual is holding his or her body in relation to the Earth and how much is in the stomach. If the person's upper body is vertical or perpendicular (i.e., sitting upright, standing) to the planet, the force of gravity will likely keep the food in the antrum or the lower part of the stomach and away from the LES and the esophagus. And if the stomach is not too full, the contents will, in most cases, stay down due to gravity.

But changing position to a more parallel or horizontal position (i.e., reclining or lying flat) may cause gravity to work against the digestive process. In these positions, the LES may be lower than the contents of the stomach. With a weakened LES, this allows the food that is consumed and the acid and enzymes that are produced in the stomach to flow into the esophagus.

Because of the potential for reflux given these dynamics, many patients find more comfort in sleeping a) at least four hours after their last bite is consumed and b) with their head and torso slightly elevated. The former suggestion is to allow the stomach enough time to digest the food and clear it from the stomach; the latter allows the stomach to work with gravity to prevent reflux.

The digestion schedule may require a little tinkering in your day to come up with the best times and the proper amounts to eat. If you regularly don't eat much of a breakfast or a lunch and come home from work famished at 8 P.M. before dropping into bed two hours later, you may want to rethink that habit. Eating a larger breakfast with less at each meal as the day progresses permits the calories to be utilized earlier in the day and the bulk of the food to be digested by bedtime. Also, it allows the body to be vertical during digestion, giving gravity an opportunity to work its magic.

When the food has digested and bedtime has arrived, reclining flat on a bed may sound comfortable but may actually cause pain in the long run. Instead, a lot of people with reflux find they can sleep through the night by raising the head of the bed by six to eight inches. This can be done a few ways. If you sleep alone or if your sleeping partner doesn't mind, you can raise the whole head of the bed by placing it on a sturdy riser, such wooden or cement blocks secured to the bed frame with rope or bungee cords; some specialty companies manufacture special cone-shaped, sturdy risers that attach to the feet of the bed and raise the bed in varying degrees. The securing of the bed frame to the risers is critical as it prevents the bed from slipping back to a level position in the middle of the night. Another important consideration is the type of sheets used when the bed is placed at such an angle. Using fine cotton with a high thread count or satin sheets can provide a slippery surface, leaving the bed's occupants to slide toward the floor. Using lower thread count sheets, cotton blends, or flannel sheets as well as placing a terry-cloth towel under the lower back and buttocks can prevent such slippage.

Patti, an interior decorator, said she often wondered why a certain client's bed skirt didn't fit quite right until the client told her that the bed was raised to avoid nighttime reflux, making the skirt gap at the head and bunch at the foot. Patti soon adapted this practice for herself, propping herself up at an angle to quell the burning pain in her throat.

Some patients find that raising the entire head of the bed is not a feasible or comfortable option. For these individuals, a wedge-shaped pillow can help to accomplish the same goal without disturbing the angle of the bed. Available in various shapes, sizes, and firmnesses, these pillows can be found at medical supply stores.

Kathy uses one of those pillows and has found it to be a tremendous help. "I purchased a Med-Slant pillow, which is used on top of the mattress, and raises my upper body by about six inches," she said. "This has been one of the most helpful things for me. It travels well, too."

A third, much more expensive option, is to buy or rent an adjustable bed, the head of which can be raised at the push of a button. Some of these beds can cost thousands of dollars; in some cases, all or a portion of the cost of the bed or rental may be covered by insurance plans.

Changing meals

EATING, FOR SOME, precipitates reflux. Whenever these individuals consume anything, the pain seems to begin. At times, people with reflux avoid eating or stick to an entirely bland menu in order to avoid any possible reaction with food.

In order to avoid the pain and the regurgitation of acid to her palate, Patrice began to shirk eating most foods, especially her morning coffee that made her retch. She skittishly tried seemingly innocuous comfort foods like soup or mashed potatoes only to find that certain ingredients would kick off a rip-roaring reflux event. She found that eating turkey sandwiches—no mustard or mayo, thanks, and skip the cheese and tomato—would be okay as would be a plain baked potato. On this diet, she dropped pounds quickly.

But humans need to eat not only for nutritional but also for social value. Foods are served for religious events, family reunions, birthdays, secular holidays, and a number of other social gatherings. We eat together as families for regular meals, as business people at dinners to close a deal, as friends catching up on the latest gossip. Often, foods are associated with memories as well. You may not remember the dress Aunt Mary wore to the family picnic, but you surely remember—even crave—her potato salad or apple pie just from a memory. To shirk food is to shirk the essence of life.

TIPS FOR CHANGING MEALS

1. Eat more but smaller meals, with most of your calories consumed by the early afternoon.
2. Control portion sizes, splitting larger meals by two or three.
3. Lower fat content in portions.
4. Cut caffeine.
5. Find out which foods are your triggers and eliminate them or find substitutes.

With reflux, many people have to relearn not only how to eat but what to eat. Life can still be enjoyed to its fullest and food can still retain much but perhaps different flavor; alterations should be made to accomplish just that.

More but smaller meals can make a huge difference in eating with reflux. The bigger the meal, the more distended the stomach is and the more work it has to do to clear itself of its contents, leading some to a nasty bout of reflux. In the same vein, eating three large meals a day may fulfill your caloric needs but so, too, will five smaller meals. Instead of having breakfast, lunch, and dinner, switch to having a smaller breakfast, a small mid-morning snack, lunch, a mid-afternoon snack, and a smaller dinner. Eating more often in the day also keeps metabolism at a steady rate.

Controlling portion size is equally important in making the switch to more but smaller meals. In this world of super sizing, meal portions served in restaurants are often three to four times the amount that should be consumed at one sitting. According to the United States Department of Agriculture's Dietary Guidelines for Americans, a single super-sized meal at a popular fast food restaurant contains nearly all of the fat and sodium, half of the protein, and almost half of the calories that dietitians suggest be consumed in an entire day. There are many strategies to combat the clean plate mindset that can make multiple meals and super sizing a potential for poundage. In many restaurants, it is perfectly acceptable to take home what is not eaten, split a meal with a fellow diner, or request half portions. If none of these are appealing, leave the leftover food and walk away from the table. Most likely, no one is forcing you to eat it all, and if they try, ignore them.

Lowering the amount of fat that is consumed in each meal will also go a long way in controlling reflux symptoms. Fat, while prompting peristaltic waves, takes longer to move through the stomach as it is more difficult to digest, thereby slowing gastric motility in many individuals. Avoiding higher-fat red meat; substituting fried selections for those that are baked, broiled, or boiled; and opting for lower-fat snacks as opposed to the full-fat varieties can go along way in reducing symptoms.

Dairy products in particular can be a cause of concern for people with reflux, as many of the popular selections such as cheese or milk are high in fat and not as easily tolerated. Additionally, dairy products are rich in calcium, a mineral that can prompt the release of hydrochloric acid in the stomach. Some people find relief from their reflux symptoms simply by ridding their diet of dairy products. Still others discover it is nearly impossible for them to do so, opting instead to limit the amount of dairy they consume and reducing the fat in their dairy choices. But switching from regular cream cheese to the fat-free variety can be like tasting paste for some, while those who drink two percent milk may feel like they are swallowing colored water when they opt for skim. To ease the transition, it may help to dilute the two percent with the skim until the taste buds adjust, just as switching to a lower-fat cheese before moving to a fat-free variety can help to bridge the gap during the adjustment phase. Still more people opt to use soy or rice milk or faux dairy tofu products. There are many tasty varieties out there, including Westsoy's Smart Lite in vanilla and the Tofutti products, especially the positively addictive ice cream sandwiches called Tofutti Cuties.

COMMON REFLUX FOOD TRIGGERS

1. Citrus foods (limes, lemons, grapefruits, oranges)
2. Acidic fruits and vegetables (tomatoes, cranberries, pineapple, cucumbers)
3. Certain vinegars and vinegar-cured condiments and foods (sauerkraut, certain olives and pickles, certain mustards)
4. Fatty or fried foods
5. Dairy products, especially those that are higher in fat content or are acidic (yogurt, for instance)
6. Hot peppers
7. Sugary treats
8. Chocolate
9. Peppermint
10. Caffeine
11. Alcohol
12. Carbonated beverages

Another area of concern in people with reflux is caffeine, a substance known to weaken the LES. Losing the caffeine can be a difficult proposition in a country where coffee shops abound and caffeinated beverages are more readily available sometimes than water. Often, eliminating caffeine can also lead to nausea and headaches. To do so with the least amount of pain, it can be beneficial to slowly lessen the amount of caffeine consumed. For example, if you are used to drinking three cups of coffee a day, try drinking two regular cups and substitute the third with a tasty herbal or decaffeinated tea, continually reducing the amount of the caffeinated beverage until it is eliminated and a substitution has been made. Other safe beverages that can be substituted for the offending caffeinated ones include milk, water, and decaffeinated or herbal teas; water is particularly useful as it helps to dilute the hydrochloric acid present in the stomach. Citrus juices such as orange, tomato, and lemonade, contain citric acid and should be avoided; however, other juices and nectars containing pears, peaches, and papayas can be more easily tolerated. Finally, decaffeinated carbonated beverages such as ginger ale are often associated with belching but may be more tolerable when they are flatter and less fizzy.

Avoiding citrus foods seems to be a given as they often contain high amounts of citric acid, potentially exacerbating reflux symptoms. But people often mistakenly think that all fruits must be avoided. In fact, some fruits can have a beneficial effect on reflux. Ripe mango and papaya, for example, tend to be more alkaline than acidic in nature. Also, the papaya contains papain, an enzyme that can help to break down protein in the stomach. Other less acidic fruits include figs, dates, ripe bananas, persimmons, peaches, pears, guava, cherries, and certain melons, such as cantaloupe.

Individuals with erosive esophagitis may find that certain peppers or pepper-containing foods may kick the taste up a notch—but also the pain. That is because certain peppers contain varying amounts of capsaicin, an oily substance that gives peppers their scorching attributes. While some peppers and pepper products—such as bell peppers—are mild, others have the intensity to burn skin. Not all peppers were created equally, however. The intensity of the burn is rated in Scoville units, the higher the rating the more potent the pepper; for example, Tabasco sauce and cayenne rate in the 30,000 to 50,000 range, serrano at 5,000 to 15,000, jalapeno at 5,000, and mild bell peppers at 0. Imagine that effect on an already burned esophagus and you will see why some doctors tell their patients to forgo peppers altogether. If you are really into peppers, you may want to try those that have a lower Scoville rating. Black pepper, the table spice, almost universally causes problems and should be avoided if that is the case.

If giving up coffee, tea, citrus foods, and other acidic foods is too much, you may want to try some commercial products that promise to reduce the amount of acid in these foods. Tamer and Preleif are both products available on the Internet or in pharmacies that can be used with these foods with varying success.

Some also avoid the so-called gassy vegetables such as broccoli, leeks, cauliflower, beans, and cabbage, as they say these will cause gas and therefore more belching. However, much of the gas that is produced from these vegetables is produced by the bacteria in the colon, the location of which precludes the notion that the gas will migrate back to the stomach and place pressure on the LES. While you may experience a little more anal wind by eating these items, you will likely not have more reflux as a result of consuming these nutrient-packed items. That said, those with gastroparesis may find it difficult to stomach these items and therefore find it wise to avoid them.

One other general category of foods that cause a problem for some are those that have a high level of sugar or are intensely sweet. Sugar in baking and cooking acts like an acid, cutting the fat in some instances in the same way that vinegar cuts the oil in salad dressings. While many people are able to tolerate the roll part of a cinnamon roll, for example, they may feel a fiery reaction to the sugar-based icing on top of it. If this proves to be impossible, limit your consumption to a bite or two of the desired goodies or consume them earlier in the day when you will likely not be reclining.

In particular, chocolate and peppermint are often served at the end of the meal, either as a dessert or as a palate cleanser. The problem with these foods in people with reflux is that their consumption often leads to an episode as they weaken the LES. And yet, it just may be darn near impossible to drop these tasty treats altogether. Again, if you can't escape the pull of these two foods, it might be best to consume them earlier in the day when you are more likely to remain upright during digestion rather than at night when they are more likely to keep you awake.

Finding a new way of dressing the salad might be important to those who experience heartburn or other reflux symptoms when they consume something as seemingly benign as tossed salad. Salad dressings often incorporate fat in the form of oil as well as garlic and other pungent spices to enhance the taste of the vegetables. Choosing a lower-fat oil such as canola or a more mild-tasting dressing can ease symptoms. To cut the oil, vinegar or citrus juices are often used in the dressings as well. We have already highlighted citrus foods, but vinegar can also cause problems as it can be highly acidic and add insult to injury in the presence of erosive esophagitis. There are at least two ways of mitigating the vinegar: Reduce the amount of vinegar or use a type of vinegar with lower acidity. Often, vinegar in salad dressing can be reduced significantly when palatable spices such as dill are introduced. Also, it is important to note that vinegars come in various acidity levels, the percentage of which are listed on the labels. For example, some balsamic vinegars register at 6 percent acidity while white wine vinegars can be 5 percent and some rice wine vinegars come in at 4.3 percent, so substituting the lower acidity vinegars can be an option for some.

WHEN TRAVELING OR EATING OUT

WHEN YOU CAN'T control your food choices is generally when trouble has the greatest chance of entering the picture. While traveling, eating out, or being entertained by others, food is generally served to you, leaving you few choices to guarantee a heartburn-free experience.

In restaurants, take care in thoroughly reading the menu and in asking questions about how the food is prepared and what ingredients are included. Don't be afraid to ask if you can make a substitution due to a health condition; most chefs are more than happy to accommodate you. Almost all restaurants will likely have at least one thing you can eat as almost every culture uses either rice or noodles as the basis of many dishes. Ask that sauces be placed on the side and that no oils or potentially harsh spices or seasonings, such as black pepper or garlic, be used in the preparation of the dish. If a particular dish includes a protein such as chicken that is sautéed or fried, ask that the chicken be grilled or broiled plain instead. Request that vegetables be cooked or steamed without oils.

While traveling, bring your own bottled water or request bottled water instead of carbonated or caffeinated beverages. If a meal is to be served in transit, find out ahead of time what choices are available. If the food selections will likely trigger a reflux episode, bring a bag of pretzels or baked potato chips to tide you over until you are able to eat a more nourishing meal. It is better to forgo the reflux trigger than to suffer in a cramped seat or, worse, retching in an airline bathroom at ten thousand feet for the next two hours.

If you have been invited to an event, it is perfectly acceptable to phone the host ahead of time and ask what will be served, being sure to cite your health concern as your reason for inquiring. Plenty of people—from those with diabetes to those with celiac sprue, from those with a heart condition to those with food allergies—have valid reasons for wanting to know what fare will be available. If the food choice is something that is sure to spoil your evening—say cream of tomato soup served with sautéed scallops drenched in a garlic butter sauce—you have three choices: decline the invitation, eat beforehand and push the food around your plate when it arrives, or offer to bring your own food and have the chef place it on a plate to be served with the other meals. The third option, as odd as it sounds, is generally the best as it accommodates your needs, allows you to attend the event, and frees the host to worry about other details than your personal needs.

Finally, there may be days when you simply cannot seem to take a bite of anything without having a reflux reaction. On days like this, it may be best to stick to safe foods such as nonfat pretzels, plain bagels, oatmeal, nonsugary cereal, simple broth, baked turkey or chicken, and other bland items. Be sure to drink plenty of water as it helps to dilute the acid in the stomach. With proper treatment and time, this episode, too, will likely pass and you will be back to eating relatively normally.

4

~~~~~

MEDICAL MANAGEMENT

In many diseases, the first line of defense often is medical treatment. Think pills, potions, and prescriptions and you are thinking medical treatments. Medications can be altered by their dosage and have a transient effect without creating lasting change to the body. They can be changed when they don't work to expectation or added to achieve the desired result. The reason that surgical intervention is seen as a last resort is because such treatment involves anesthesia, cutting, pain, long healing times, possible complications, and greater costs, consequences that may possibly be avoided by simply swallowing a pill or more a day.

The goals of medical treatment for GERD include reducing and eliminating the symptoms caused by the reflux, primarily through controlling acid production or by moving food and beverages more quickly through the upper digestive system. In those with erosive esophagitis, the added goal is the healing of the esophagus through initial treatment and maintenance therapy, a sustained therapy that continues after healing to prevent new damage. For patients with symptoms that occur while sleeping, another goal is to eliminate nocturnal symptoms through acid suppression. In any case, the treatment can take a few weeks to several months and may have to be repeated as the condition resurfaces.

The type of treatment that is prescribed is based on the severity of the symptoms and the results of the tests described in the previous chapter. For those with mild and infrequent heartburn symptoms, common remedies found on the shelves of the local drugstore will likely be all that is needed. Conversely, those with more severe and persistent symptoms or those who fail to achieve results with the more mild medications require more comprehensive treatment involving lifestyle modification and a more potent drug to battle back to a sense of normalcy.

While no one really relishes swallowing medication on a regular basis, the good news is that doctors have come a long way in understanding the mechanisms of acid production and therefore have developed effective means of treating GERD. In the last century, dozens of medications to treat GERD—from gentle over-the-counter **antacids** and **histamine H$_2$ blockers** to the more powerful prescription **prokinetic agents** and **proton pump inhibitors**—have been created and used with varying levels of success. It seems as though new, more effective, treatments make their debut each year and are more competent at forcing some of the most stubborn cases of GERD into silence.

It is important to note here the therapies listed below do not cure GERD, as there is no cure for the disease at this time. Instead, these medications are used to help control the symptoms and allow healing to occur. It is also essential to understand that you should consult your physician before taking any medication, even the over-the-counter variety. Your physician should be aware of your physical changes, even seemingly innocuous ones.

ANTACIDS AND ACID-REDUCTION MEDICATIONS AND HOW THEY WORK

Antacids

Antacids, in many different forms, have been in use for several centuries and are quite common in Western culture, at least a portion of the population of which can likely recite any number of different advertising jingles for these products. "Plop, plop, fizz, fizz. Oh, what a relief it is!" "Tums, Tums, Tums, Tums, Tums." "I can't believe I ate the whole thing."

Aside from the catchy slogans, the products are popular because they generally act quickly to neutralize the acidity of the stomach contents. Acidity is based on the **pH scale,** which begins at zero and runs to fourteen, with a score in the middle being neutral. The lower the number is below seven, the more acidic the object is; conversely, the higher the number is above seven, the more alkaline the object is. The contents of the stomach, which is built to withstand low acid counts, are usually about a two or three on the pH scale. In the esophagus, the mucosa is more sensitive and best able to handle a four or higher.

On the basic level, the antacids work to bring the acidity to a more comfortable five or above. With the addition of certain ingredients, some products also form a comforting foamy barrier on the top of the gastric pool (alginic acid) while others help to contain gas bubbles from resulting in a burp that can heave the acidic gastric contents into the esophagus (simethicone). Antacids also come in a variety of forms, from gel caps to chewable tablets to liquids, and are generally affordable to the average consumer. Usually, these medications are used for occasional GERD, such as when you indulge a bit too much on the burritos and margaritas.

There are primarily four main ingredients in antacids. In alphabetical order, they are:

- Aluminum salts, such as aluminum hydroxide, aluminum phosphate gel, and aluminum carbonate, are other common ingredients in antacids. In addition to causing constipation in some individuals, long-term use of medications containing this ingredient cause the leaching of calcium, phosphates, and fluorides from the bones, causing them to weaken.

- Calcium carbonate or calcium phosphate, referred to as calcium salts, also are common ingredients in certain antacids. Calcium carbonate is also commonly used in calcium supplements such as Caltrate and OsCal as well as the popular antacid Tums. Though they are effective in neutralizing the stomach acid and can boost a diet flagging in calcium, they also carry with them the less-than-desirable side effect of constipation in some individuals. Excessive calcium can lead to the formation of painful kidney stones.

- Magnesium salts in different incarnations—carbonate, hydroxide, aluminosilicates, to name a few—also act quickly to neutralize acid and are often mixed with at least one of the other three ingredients to offset a laxative effect that naturally accompanies it. Too much of the medication can cause problems with the heart and kidneys while long-term use of the drug can cause kidney stones in some individuals.

- Sodium bicarbonate, more commonly known as baking soda, has many uses outside of an ingredient in antacids. Mixed with a bit of water to make a paste, it can take the sting out of an insect bite or a burn. In bathwater, it can soothe a case of the hives. On a toothbrush, it can substitute for toothpaste. In antacids, the sodium bicarbonate acts quickly to neutralize the existing stomach acid, usually in a fizzy form such as in Alka Seltzer or Bromo Seltzer. This medication is not for all GERD patients as it contains sodium and can interfere with a low-sodium diet.

All antacids can interfere with the absorption of certain medications or decrease their effectiveness. Also, some individuals taking antacids experience acid rebound, a condition marked by an initial decrease in acidity that is followed by an increase in acid levels, leaving some physicians to shy away from recommending them in the first place. Side effects of some antacids include increased thirst and abdominal cramps. Because of this, it is wise to consult a doctor before ingesting them.

The upside of taking an antacid is that the action is very close to immediate, taming the acidity in a matter or minutes. Aside from the possibility of acid rebound, the downside of taking antacids is that they are short-lived in nature and not a good option for those who are struggling with a more active case of GERD.

Histamine H$_2$ Blockers

The release of different histamines in the body causes a slew of different reactions such as allergic reactions and secretion of hydrochloric acid in the stomach for digestion. The latter is of concern in relation to GERD.

The theory behind the class of drugs known as histamine H$_2$ blockers (also known as H$_2$ receptor antagonists or H$_2$RAs) goes like this: When the histamine is released during digestion, it has to be received, the action of which prompts the release of the hydrochloric acids. By entering the bloodstream and blocking the receptors, the drugs cut the chain reaction short, thus suppressing the production of acid.

When the histamine H$_2$ blockers were first introduced in the 1970s, they were purely prescription drugs. However, drug companies were able to gain approval of over-the-counter formulations in lower doses in the 1990s, making them more easily accessible. As a general rule, prescription-strength drugs have twice or more the strength of over-the-counter drugs. For a mild or occasional case of GERD, a physician may first recommend the over-the-counter formulation before moving to a prescription-strength formulation. Also, the drugs can be used in conjunction with proton pump inhibitors for stubborn cases of GERD but should not be taken within an hour of taking an antacid due to the decreased effectiveness that may result. That said, some over-the-counter formulations such as Pepcid Complete contain both antacids (calcium carbonate and magnesium hydrochloride) and an H$_2$ blocker. The drugs, marketed to those with mild to moderate GERD, come in different flavors, from cherry to mint, and in different forms, including pills, chewables, liquids, and effervescents.

Currently, there are four major drugs that fall into this category. In alphabetical order, they are:

■ ■ ■

- Cimetidine (Tagamet line of products) is used by individuals who seek to control GERD as well as by those who are trying to allow a stomach or duodenal ulcer to heal or those with Zollinger-Ellison syndrome who are trying to control acid. For those with reflux and erosive esophagitis, the usual prescription dose for the light green 200, 300, 400, and 800 mg tablets is 1,600 mgs a day either taken in two 800 mg doses or four 400 mg doses for twelve weeks; the medication also comes in a peach-mint flavored syrup and by injection. For those using the over-the-counter formulation Tagamet HB, the usual dose is two tablets twice a day, but no more than four tablets a day. Individuals with liver or kidney disease should discuss taking cimetidine with their doctor. Also, there is a fair list of medications such as the blood thinner Coumadin, antibiotics such as metronidazole (Flagyl) and amoxicillin with clavulanate (Augmentin), beta blockers, and antidepressants with which the drug can have adverse reactions or can affect the efficacy, so it is important to discuss with the doctor all medications that are taken before taking the drug. The side effects include breast development in men, headaches, agitation, anxiety, and depression.

- By prescription, famotidine (Mylanta AR, Pepcid line of products), used by the same population as those who use cimetidine, comes in disintegrating tablets and as beige tablets and brownish-orange tablets in doses of 20 mgs and 40 mgs; an oral suspension formula is available as well. For use in reflux, the dosage guidelines suggest that the usual dose is 20 mgs or 2.5 milliliters twice a day for six weeks, up to twice that amount if erosive esophagitis exists for twice the duration. A word to the wise: The medication that dissolves in the mouth can leave a chalky residue behind. The medication should be used with caution by those with kidney disease since the medication is excreted from the body through the kidneys. Also, those on the antifungal drugs Sporanox or Nizoral should consult their doctors regarding usage and potential counteractions.

- Nizatidine (Axid line of products) is also used in the same population as the above drugs. The usual prescription dosage of the drug is 150 mgs, twice a day; the capsules are dark and light yellow. Usually, the drug is not taken for longer than eight weeks unless used as maintenance therapy in certain individuals; in those cases, the drug is taken at lower doses. A doctor should be notified if moderate to severe kidney disease exists or if aspirin is taken on a regular basis. The common side effects of the drug include gastrointestinal upset such as nausea, pain, diarrhea, or gas, as well as dizziness, sore throat, inflammation of the nose, and weakness.

- Ranitidine hydrochloride (Zantac line of products) is also used in the same patient population as the other histamine H_2 blockers. The drug is available in a wide array of forms—from injection to effervescent tablets, from peppermint-flavored syrup to peach-colored tablets—and in different dosage levels as well. The drug is also one of the only reflux drugs to be tested in the pediatric population (see chapter 7). For reflux, the usual daily dose is 150 mgs or 10 milliliters twice a day, for four to eight weeks. For reflux with erosive esophagitis, the 150 mg or 10 milliliter dose is taken four times a day, dwindling to a maintenance dose of twice a day when the damage has healed. Like cimetidine, the list of drugs with which it can have an interaction or with which it can change efficacy is long and includes sedatives like diazepam (Valium), antidiabetes drugs like glipizide (Glocotrol) and metformin (Glucophage), and antifungal drugs ketoconazole (Nizoral) and itraconazole (Sporanox), among others. The most commonly reported side effect is headache.

All of the drugs can mask the presence of a stomach malignancy even if the histamine H_2 blockers relieve the symptoms, which is why it is important to be thoroughly checked by a physician before taking the medication. The upside of taking the blockers is that they work to stop the production of the acid for several hours, not merely tame it for a short time. Therefore, the results are longer lasting than with an antacid. However, the downside is that they must first enter the bloodstream before they can work, leaving a forty-minute to one-hour span before relief comes. In the case of anticipating heartburn due to a potentially reflux-inducing meal, it is wise to take the medication before sitting down to the table.

Proton pump inhibitors

The newest kid on the block, the proton pump inhibitors (PPI) debuted in the late 1980s and early 1990s to great fanfare. The drugs were touted as being more effective then the histamine H_2 blockers as well as being effective in healing erosive esophagitis and controlling symptoms in those with moderate to severe GERD. Prescriptions were written by the millions, despite a monthly cost of about $120, a hardship for those with no or insufficient prescription insurance coverage.

Like the histamine H_2 blockers, the proton pump inhibitors, once ingested, must enter the blood stream to provide relief. Once in the blood, they travel to the hydrogen-potassium adenosine triphosphate enzyme system, a large name for a tiny mechanism that is located on the surface of the gastric parietal cell. There, they bond with the proton pumps to inactivate them for twenty-four to seventy-two hours. By doing this, the drug acts to immobilize the very mechanism that produces the hydrochloric acid in the stomach.

A number of similar proton pump inhibitors have flooded the market in the past decade. Each of the drugs has been shown in several studies to be effective. All carry about the same wholesale price, ranging from $3 to $4 for the daily dose. All are used in the treatment of symptomatic GERD and erosive esophagitis as well as serving as a maintenance therapy for those with healing or healed erosive esophagitis. Additionally, the drugs are used to treat gastric or duodenal ulcers and hypersecretory conditions such as Zollinger-Ellison syndrome.

In alphabetical order, the PPIs include:

- Lansoprazole (Prevacid), in pink and green or pink and black capsules, comes in 15 mg or 30 mg doses and is available in oral suspension packets that can be mixed with water. The usual daily dose for symptomatic GERD is 15 mg once daily; and for erosive esophagitis is 30 mgs once daily; maintenance therapy can continue at 15 mgs. Because lansoprazole suppresses acid production, as do all PPIs, it can interfere with the absorption of medications that rely on acidity to break them down, such as ketoconazole (Nizoral), iron supplements, and ampicillin esters (Omnipen or Principen). For those who have difficulty swallowing pills, the contents of the lansoprazole capsule can be mixed with applesauce and ingested instead.

- Omeprazole (Prilosec) and esomeprazole (Nexium) are grouped together because a) they are made by the same pharmaceutical company, AstraZeneca and b) esomeprazole is a close cousin to the original omeprazole, the first PPI approved for use in the United States. Omeprazole, in apricot and amethyst or amethyst capsules, is generally prescribed in 20 milligram doses, once a day for four to eight weeks and sometimes longer as a maintenance therapy; the drug is available in 10 mg, 20 mg, and 40 mg dosages. The drug was released for sale in 2003 as an over-the-counter formulation, which means that you don't have to have a prescription to get it. The pills come in 20 milligram doses and are to be taken once a day for a 14-day course, no more than one course in four months. Esomeprazole comes in 20 mg and 40 mg purple capsules to be taken once daily and can be taken for the same amount of time. For erosive esophagitis, the drug can be continued for maintenance therapy following healing. The drugs can cause an alteration in the metabolism of diazepam (Valium), warafin (Coumadin), and phenytoin (Dilantin) and there have been clinical reports regarding altered absorption of cyclosporine (Sandimmune, Neoral), disulfiram (Antabuse), and benzodiazepines, as well as ketoconazole (Nizoral), certain iron supplements, and ampicillin esters (Omnipen or Principen). The medications should be taken about an hour before eating. Like lansoprazole, esomeprazole capsules can be broken open and the contents mixed with cold applesauce.

- Pantoprazole (Protonix) comes in 40 mg yellow tablets and in an intravenous formulation for those who cannot take tablets. The daily dose for erosive esophagitis is 40 mg taken once daily for up to eight weeks or longer for maintenance therapy. Pantoprazole does not have the documented side effects and drug interactions that omeprazole does but essentially has the same side effects and drug interactions as lansoprazole. The drug cannot be crushed for those with swallowing difficulties, as the enteric coating should remain intact until after the drug leaves the stomach.

- Rabeprazole (AcipHex) comes in 20 mg enteric-coated pale yellow tablets that should not be chewed, smashed, or broken before ingesting them; the pills are smaller than the rest of the PPIs and therefore may be easier to swallow. For GERD and the healing of erosive esophagitis, the medication is taken at 20 mg once a day for eight weeks or longer as a maintenance therapy. The drug can affect the absorption of medications that rely on acidity to break them down such as ketoconazole (Nizoral), iron supplements, and ampicillin esters (Omnipen or Principen) and has had an effect on the absorption of cyclosporine (Sandimmune and Neoral) and digoxin (Lanoxin).

For the most part, the drugs enter the bloodstream and travel to the liver where they are metabolized by different enzymes. Because everyone has different body chemistry, certain PPIs may be more effective than others due to the differences in the enzymatic action. For example, certain studies show that pantoprazole, omeprazole, esomeprazole and, to a certain extent, lansoprazole are metabolized by a certain enzyme that may be lacking in portions of the Caucasian and Asian population and thus would not be as effective as other PPIs. Therefore, a doctor may go through a few PPIs before finding the right one for a patient.

All of the drugs come in different dosing levels, allowing a little leverage for the physician in prescribing. Also, some come in different forms, such as in oral suspension packets for adults or liquid suspension for children (lansoprazole comes in both forms), while others are available in intravenous preparations (pantoprazole) for those who are unable to take the oral dosages. In a number of different trials, the drugs were comparatively the same in side effects reported, including headache, nausea, vomiting, diarrhea, and abdominal pain.

Though only one of these drugs is available over the counter, more will likely follow suit in the years to come, thus providing a more affordable and convenient option for those without prescription drug insurance coverage.

■   ■   ■

FOR SOME INDIVIDUALS, the medications designed as antacids and acid suppressors are enough in that the drugs can help them to control their symptoms while allowing those with a damaged esophagus to heal properly. But others may require a little more help pharmaceutically, with what are known as complementary therapies, medications taken in addition to the main medication that can help to control some of the manifestations or potential causes of GERD.

Prokinetic agents

Some patients find that the food they have eaten takes longer to leave the stomach than is usual, a condition known as delayed gastric emptying or slow gastric motility. When this occurs, it leaves a longer window of opportunity for the acid to rise in the esophagus. For these patients, it may be helpful if they combine anti-reflux therapy with medication designed to empty the stomach more expeditiously.

Called prokinetic medication, these drugs work to move food and beverages along at a swifter pace through the esophagus and the stomach while also having the possible added benefit in some individuals of strengthening the LES. Often, these medications are used for those with gastroparesis.

One such medication in GERD is metoclopramide hydrochloride (Reglan), which comes in the forms of injection, tablet, or syrup. The drug may be used in 10 to 15 mg doses four times a day or as symptoms occur.

The side effects reported in this class of drug include drowsiness or fatigue; in some individuals, restlessness in the form of jumpiness, nervousness, or spastic movements of limbs can also occur. Some individuals with Parkinson's disease report a worsening of symptoms. Additionally, the drug can interact with other medications including, but not limited to, certain antidepressants, narcotic painkillers, tranquilizers, and sleeping pills, so it is important to discuss with the doctor all medications that are being used in conjunction with the prokinetic agents. Because these side effects are often not well tolerated, this drug is not commonly used.

There are two other drugs that deserve to be mentioned, even if they are not currently available in the United States. Domperidone (Motilium) is a prokinetic drug that is currently available in Canada and Europe and that reportedly has fewer side effects than metoclopramide hydrochloride. Cisapride (Propulsid) was originally approved for use in the United States by the FDA. However, documented cases of heart rhythm abnormalities, some of which lead to death of the users, led the manufacturer to pull the drug from the shelves in 1999. It is available now only in limited prescriptions through the government.

Depending on the symptoms that the person with GERD experiences, different medications can be helpful as well. For example, a small portion of GERD patients complain of difficulty breathing, possibly due in part to acid that is breathed into the airways and causes irritation in the pulmonary system. For these patients, certain medications used to make breathing easier in people with asthma, such as bronchodilators, can help. In others who experience a sore throat, something as simple as over-the-counter acetaminophen (Tylenol) can be taken to ease the pain.

MEDICATIONS THAT CAN HURT

NOT ALL MEDICATIONS are created equally. That said, some medications that produce a positive effect on certain diseases might worsen a case of heartburn.

Anticholinergic agents

Just as prokinetic agents act on the nerve responses in the upper gastrointestinal system to quickly move stomach contents into the intestines, there are other drugs that can have the opposite effect. Anticholinergic agents are prescribed for a number of conditions in which spasms in the muscles cause discomfort. For example, the drugs are used to control tremors in Parkinson's disease. The drugs are also prescribed for irritable bowel syndrome, a frequently misunderstood condition that causes abdominal pain, diarrhea, constipation, or both, in some individuals. Commonly prescribed anticholinergics for the bowels include dicyclomine (Bentyl) and L-hyoscyamine (Levsin).

While they can stop a case of diarrhea on a dime, the slowing of the bowels can mean a more slowly emptying stomach as well, leading to a possible increase in GERD symptoms.

Calcium channel blockers

These kinds of medications, including diltiazem (Cardizem) and nifedipine (Procardia), are widely used in the treatment of heart disease and high blood pressure. In these diseases, the drugs act to keep calcium in heart and blood vessel cells static and relax the smooth muscles cells in the process. This action allows for a greater movement of blood and oxygen through the cardiovascular system.

While it works wonders in that application, this class of drugs can increase the incidence of GERD in some individuals. This is because the smooth muscle cells exist in the gastrointestinal system as well. Making those cells more static means slowing the system's movements, theoretically leaving food to sit in the stomach for longer periods of time and potentially opening the door to greater reflux symptoms.

Barbiturates and narcotic analgesics

Barbiturates are sedatives that are commonly used to allay anxiety, ward off seizures, and allow for sleep in insomniacs. Narcotic analgesics are medications that employ opium or opium derivatives to relieve intense pain. Both classes of drugs act on the central nervous system to slow heart rate, blood pressure, and temperature.

While a godsend to those who need them for various conditions, the drugs can act to slow the gastrointestinal tract in many of those who take them, having an effect similar to anticholinergic agents in those with GERD.

Nicotine and alcohol

Nicotine and alcohol are perhaps the most commonly ingested over-the-counter drugs in America. According to a Centers for Disease Control study, about one in four Americans smoke. Other studies find that nearly 70 percent of Americans drink one to two alcoholic beverages a week.

While a beer and a smoke may be just the ticket for some who strive to relax, those with GERD would be wise to avoid either or the combination. Both alcohol and nicotine serve to reduce pressure in the LES, potentially leading to greater heartburn in those who imbibe. In addition, alcohol contains empty calories, potentially leading to a weight gain that can also lead to a higher rate of reflux in some.

Non-steroidal anti-inflammatory drugs (NSAID)

NSAIDs are common medications found on the shelves of every pharmacy in America. Ibuprofen (Advil, Motrin), aspirin (Bayer), ketoprofen (Orudis), and naproxen (Naprosyn, Aleve) are all used to cut pain and inflammation quickly.

But while these are favored medications of many people, the medications are known to cause gastrointestinal bleeding and ulceration in many individuals, conditions that can complicate healing of erosive esophagitis or irritate an already raging case of GERD. Due to this, it might be better to stick to the acetaminophen concentrations that are also on the market.

■ ■ ■

TIPS FOR TAKING MEDICATION

YOU COULD have the best, most powerful medication in the world to stop heartburn, but it isn't going to work if you don't take it properly and consistently. Remembering to take your medication and making it a part of your everyday routine can be a challenge, even for the most organized among us. The following are some tips for making pill taking easier:

- Some medication must be taken with food or before you eat, especially with the histamine H_2 blockers. Since hunger rarely befalls us suddenly, remind yourself to take your medication as you prepare your food or prepare to sit down to eat.

- Look to mealtimes and bedtimes as the times to take your medication. Since few of us skip meals and all of us have to sleep, these are ideal daily times to take your medication.

- If you use a day planner, write in the times to take medication and keep handy a list of medication that has to be taken and at what times. If you are particularly bad at remembering your medication, employ others to help you through phone calls or gentle reminders.

- Making sure your medication is visible is also an easy way to remember to take it. Although you should always use care with medication around children, stashing the bottles in a drawer or a cupboard leaves them out of sight and out of mind.

- Set a day each month to refill your prescriptions, writing the number of the pharmacy directly on the calendar. On-line pharmacies are particularly helpful in this regard as they send regular E-mail messages reminding their users to reorder medication ahead of time.

- Use a pillbox that you can carry with you. Some even come with vibrating or sound alarms to remind you when to take your medication. You can get away with this option for under ten dollars, but the cost rises with the bells and whistles, literally.

- Go on-line and buy a watch with an alarm or a pill-bottle cap that contains an alarm. Program your personal computer or computerized date book to alert you when it is time to take the medication. Set your pager to go off to remind you of a dosage. Although these gadgets are

continued

great reminder tools, one obvious problem arises when the technology designed to remind us is not close at hand. The beeping pill containers, for example, could be blaring away while we run to the grocery store or the watches may be forgotten, left on the bedside table all day chirping an endless reminder that is not heard.

- If you have cash to burn and plan to be home all day, buy a dispensing machine. These gadgets, running up to one thousand dollars, must be loaded and programmed to spit out the pills at the correct time each day. They require a little know-how, so if you haven't figured out how to set the clock on your DVD player yet, it may not be a good option for you.

5

ANTIREFLUX ENDOSCOPIC AND
SURGICAL PROCEDURES

FOR THE VAST majority of people with reflux, surgery will never even enter their radar for treatment options. That fact is largely due to the innovations in treatment options that have been created in the last four decades or so, namely the histamine H_2 blockers and the PPIs discussed in the last chapter. Further understanding of the condition and its prompts has led many doctors to combine medical treatment with lifestyle modifications to bring some of the more difficult cases under control to the point where the patients do not experience symptoms. In fact, a variety of different studies point out that the current acid-reducing drugs and lifestyle modifications help to control reflux in more than 90 percent of reflux patients.

That is all well and good, unless you are in that group comprising less than 10 percent of reflux patients who don't respond to lifestyle modifications and medication or who opt not to take such steps for the rest of their lives. For some of those individuals, surgery may be their last or best chance at living a life without reflux.

■ ■ ■

Reasons for surgery and endoscopic procedures

THE REASONS FOR surgery vary from individual to individual but in general can be grouped into two categories: those for whom medical management has either failed or is too much of an onus to continue and those for whom a complication has proven too difficult to overcome with medical treatment.

Those in the first group are usually individuals who have tried all of the different medications and continue to have symptoms despite the most rigorous medical treatment available; some of these individuals seek to wean themselves from the medication after a specified period but find that the reflux usually returns with a vengeance not long after the last pill is taken. This group of patients might also include those who feel that they do not want to continue or won't be able to comply with medical orders due to an aversion to taking medication for a long time; still others may see the surgery as a less expensive option to taking pricey drugs for an extended period of time.

Those in the second group include people who have a stricture in their esophagus, commonly referred to as a "peptic stricture." Formed of scar tissue that is usually the result of repeated bouts of reflux, the strictures can at times be dilated using an inflatable balloon attachment during endoscopy or with what is known as a "bougie," a mercury-filled rubber tube that helps to expand the stricture. However, the somewhat painful procedure has to be repeated regularly in most individuals, something that is not usually relished. Another group of people in this category are those with a hiatal hernia; some of these individuals can survive well enough on medical therapy but a portion of this group is better off correcting the condition with surgery. Barrett's esophagus is often another cause for concern and a reason for surgical therapy in some individuals; however, it has not been established that antireflux surgical therapy is a means to reverse or contain Barrett's. Another subgroup of patients in this category are those who, despite the best medical treatment, continue to have extra-esophogeal conditions related to the GERD, such as wheezing, coughing, a hoarse voice, or persistent reflux-related chest pain.

Not all patients with the above reasons for antireflux surgery qualify for surgery or an endoscopic procedure, however. If a patient is not healthy enough to withstand a procedure due to other health conditions or advanced age, a doctor may not recommend it and instead continue to attempt to treat the condition medically. Also, if the normal movements of the esophagus are impaired or compromised prior to the procedure, it may actually make swallowing more difficult and cause further discomfort to the patient. Therefore, surgical and endoscopic procedures may not be recommended in patients with esophageal motility issues.

TYPES OF ANTIREFLUX SURGERY AND ENDOSCOPIC PROCEDURES

THERE EXIST SEVERAL options when it comes to antireflux surgery but all of them have the same goal: to strengthen the LES pressure to prevent the reflux of stomach contents into the esophagus. That said, each surgery is a little different, in part to care for the varying needs of the diverse reflux population. For example, there are certain surgeries that help to extend a shortened esophagus while others are more suited to the patient with a hiatal hernia in need of repair. Below are the general categories of the surgeries with an explanation of the different techniques. One important note is required here and, frankly, can not be stated enough: All surgical procedures require a skilled, experienced surgeon.

Fundoplication

The most commonly performed antireflux surgery involves the tightening of the LES by wrapping the upper portion of the stomach, the fundus, either all the way around or partially around the lower part of the esophagus and stitching it in place; the fundus then acts like a belt of sorts, cinching the LES. Called **fundoplication**, the majority of these surgeries in the past were done via an open incision in the chest or upper abdomen through which the surgery was performed. This open procedure left patients with a greater risk of postsurgical incision infection and longer healing times. Most of these procedures are now done utilizing laparoscopic techniques. Using this method, surgeons make small incisions in the upper torso through which they insert different arms of a small, endoscopic-like device called a **laparoscope**. One part of the tool inflates the cavity with carbon dioxide, allowing the surgeon to see more clearly the esophagus and the stomach. Other parts of the tool allow the surgeon to see, hold, cut, and stitch the parts of the digestive tract to complete the operation. When the operation is complete, the surgeon withdraws the tool and stitches closed the initial incisions, usually small enough to cover with a Band-Aid.

The site and type of surgery performed is dependent upon the unique circumstances that each patient presents. For those people who are overweight or obese, it may be easier for the surgeon to go through the chest or thoracic cavity rather than to attempt the same surgery through the abdomen. For those who have a short esophagus, it may be necessary to address this problem through the chest as well. But by and large, the majority of antireflux surgeries are being done through the abdomen using the laparoscope.

Within this category of antireflux surgery, there are different kinds of procedures, all named for pioneering surgeons who first performed them. Again, each surgical technique is unique and demanding, requiring a surgeon with much experience to perform it.

- Belsey fundoplication—This is one of the two most common laparoscopic techniques used in antireflux surgery. Named for British surgeon Ronald Belsey, this surgery is done through an incision in the chest wall in an open, traditional manner. During this procedure, the surgeon will wrap the fundus 270 degrees or three-quarters of the way around the esophagus. A similar variation of the procedure is known as the Belsey-Mark fundoplication. At times when the esophagus is too short, this procedure is combined with another surgical procedure known as the Collis gastroplasty, described below.
- Dor fundoplication—This surgical technique, usually performed with a laparoscope, involves wrapping the fundus 180 degrees or halfway around the anterior or front of the esophagus.
- Lind fundoplication—Another partial laparoscopic fundoplication, this procedure involves wrapping the esophagus 270 degrees or three-quarters of the way around the esophagus, covering all of the posterior or back side of the esophagus.
- Nissen fundoplication—This is one of the two most common laparoscopic techniques used in antireflux surgery. A total wrap of the esophagus, this surgery is named for Swiss surgeon Rudolf Nissen. Primarily, this surgery is performed laproscopically and can be combined with the Collis gastroplasty in certain situations in which the esophagus is shortened.

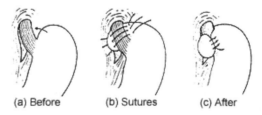

(a) Before   (b) Sutures   (c) After

FIGURE 6. NISSEN FUNDOPLICATION

Source: *Digestive Disease Dictionary,* a publicaiton of the National Institute for Diabetes, Digestive and Kidney Diseases

■ ■ ■

- Thal fundoplication—Also done laparoscopically, this wrap done on the anterior or front side of the esophagus involves 90 percent or one-quarter of the circumference of the esophagus.
- Toupet fundoplication—This laparoscopic procedure involves a wrap that involves half or a little more than half (180 to 200 degrees) of the posterior or back side of the esophagus.
- Watson fundoplication—This laparoscopic procedure involves a wrap of the front or anterior part of the esophagus by 90 to 100 degrees, or roughly one-quarter to just more than a quarter of the esophagus.

At times, a Collis **gastroplasty** is combined with one of the Fundoplication techniques to lengthen a short esophagus. Like plastic surgery for the stomach, this procedure involves the slicing of the gastric cardia in one direction, pinching the corners of the incision together and sewing it closed in the opposite direction to lengthen it. Usually, this is combined with the Belsey or Nissen fundoplication, resulting in a longer esophagus and a tighter LES.

The surgery is performed under general anesthesia and can take one to four hours to perform, depending on the skill of the surgeon and the various complications presented. Different hospitals, insurance companies, and doctors recommend different timetables for hospital stays following fundoplication surgery. For open surgery, the hospital time is usually four to six days; laparoscopic fundoplication patients usually log one to four days in the hospital.

Stretta procedure

Really considered a nonsurgical endoscopic procedure since it does not involve incisions and surgical manipulation, the **Stretta procedure** is conducted under sedation in an endoscopic suite and is considered an outpatient procedure in most cases, allowing the patient to go home in the same day.

In this procedure, the patient is sedated just as he or she would be during a normal endoscopic procedure. Then, the doctor inserts a catheter through the patient's mouth and down the esophagus to the gastroesophageal junction. Small sensors are placed in the mucosa to monitor temperature. Radio frequency waves are administered through the ball-like device at the end of the catheter, making the area hot and creating thermal lesions where coagulation of blood takes place. During the procedure, water delivered through the catheter soothes the mucosa. This process is repeated as necessary in the surrounding tissue. The device is then withdrawn and the patient is sent to recovery. In the days to come, the tissue in the gastroesophageal junction heals, albeit a bit thicker. This allows the lumen at the LES to be narrower and theoretically stronger as a result.

The procedure is relatively new, having been approved by the Food and Drug Administration (FDA) in 2000; as of the date of this publication, about three thousand such procedures had been performed internationally. Therefore, there is no data currently on the safety and long-term efficacy of the treatment. That said, the majority of the patients treated in studies submitted during the approval process received the intended benefit of the procedure.

Bard (EndoCinch) procedure

Using an endoscope, the **Bard procedure** or endoluminal gastroplication is also a noninvasive, nonsurgical technique used to strengthen the LES. The procedure requires the same sedation used during a normal endoscopic exam and allows the patient to return home hours after the procedure.

After sedating the patient, the doctor inserts into the esophagus an endoscope that has been outfitted with a special attachment that is similar to a small-scale sewing machine. Just below the LES, two stitches are placed and then drawn together, with one fold of mucosa on top of the other. This forms a sort of pleat, not unlike the pleats in a skirt or a pair of pants. By doing so, the LES is altered to make it stronger in resisting the reflux of the acidic stomach contents, and the lumen is naturally made smaller. In the Bard procedure, the initial studies submitted to the FDA for the approval process were done on a patient body that did not have hiatal hernias, motility issues, or Barrett's esophagus; because of this, some doctors are not doing that particular procedure on patients with those conditions.

Because the FDA approved this procedure in 2000, no long-term studies exist as to its relative benefit, safety, or efficacy. However, the short-term studies submitted during the FDA approval process indicate that most patients who have had the procedure done have no or mild reflux six months after the procedure and most are able to forgo or reduce their acid-reducing medications. Be that as it may, about 3,800 such procedures were done worldwide at the time of publication; because of this, many doctors are not as familiar or comfortable with the procedure and may not recommend it for their patients.

RISKS OF ANTIREFLUX SURGERY AND ENDOSCOPIC PROCEDURES

THERE ARE RISKS with any surgery. Some people can react badly to the anesthesia that is administered during the procedure while others will develop post surgical infections, despite all precautions. Still others may suffer as a result of a surgical mistake, even in the hands of a highly skilled surgeon. These risks, including a small percentage that prove fatal, are inherent in any surgical procedure, be it neuro-surgery or podiatric surgery, and antireflux surgery is no different.

All surgeries that tighten the LES carry with them additional risks and possible less-than-desirable aftereffects. For one, **gas-bloat syndrome** is reported in some patients following surgery. Because the LES is tighter than it was before, swallowed air and gasses that are created during digestion have a harder time leaving through the mouth and must travel through the digestive system to the opposite exit. This can lead to an uncomfortable experience not only socially but also physically, as being gassy can be painful to some. In the same vein, it may be more difficult to vomit as well.

Because the LES is tighter, esophageal muscles may have to work harder to move food and beverages through to the stomach. In many cases, difficulty in swallowing eases following fundoplication surgery and may be relieved by following a diet (see below) of soft foods and by chewing all foods well. In other cases, the swallowing dif-ficulty can be eased in a follow-up surgery that loosens a bit of the wrap. Also, in all upper GI endoscopic procedures, one of the risks is a sore throat for a short time after the procedure.

In any of the procedures listed above, some individuals find that the first one is not the charm. A wrap can slip or come completely undone, the stitches in the Bard procedure can come undone or not be adequate, and the thickened LES in the ini-tial Stretta procedure may not be enough. In all of these cases, a second trip to the surgeon or doctor might be required to correct the shortcoming. Don't be alarmed if this is the case, as it happens more often that one might think.

In antireflux surgical and endoscopic procedures, a patient who is a candidate should discuss the possible risks of the procedure, including the possibility that the procedure may fail and further procedures would be required. Following the procedure, all side effects or problems should be reported to the physician who performed it.

WHAT TO EXPECT FROM THE HOSPITAL EXPERIENCE AND RECOVERY

NO PERFECTLY SANE, healthy individual embraces the idea of going to a hospital, even if only to visit a sick relative or friend for an hour or two, much less to stay there for any length of time. A patient is on someone else's schedule, being poked and prod-ded on someone else's orders, and in a bed and a room not his or her own, making the experience unpredictable at best, torture at worst. Because of this, it helps to be prepared for the experience, at least mentally if not physically as well. The more you know about what to expect, the more comfortable you may be about the experience. Whatever the case, always keep this in mind: This, too, shall pass.

In any procedure to tighten the LES, the doctors and surgeons may require that certain tests be performed if they haven't been already. In particular, the esophageal manometry may be required to rule out any underlying motility disorder since tightening the LES may only exacerbate that condition. The 24-hour ambulatory pH testing may also be ordered to further assure the doctor that acid reflux is indeed the root of the problem, particularly in those who show no endoscopic sign of esophagitis. A chest Xray and preprocedure blood work will also help to guide the surgeon during the procedure and the recovery.

For those individuals who are scheduled for the Stretta or Bard procedures, the preparation is similar to the preparation for an upper GI endoscopic exam. You likely will be told to refrain from eating or drinking anything for six to eight hours before the procedure begins. You will then register, change into a hospital gown or similar garb, and be hooked up to an intravenous line. Your doctor will then greet you and discuss what will be happening next. A sedative, usually Valium, and pain medication, commonly Demerol, with an amnesia drug, Versed, will be administered to the IV line; occasionally, a short acting anesthesia, commonly Propofol, will be administered. The type of the anesthesia is usually based on any past adverse reactions you may have experienced as well as on the surgeon's proclivity for certain sedation.

When you wake up, the doctor will have performed the procedure and will soon discuss what occurred while you were out. After going over some brief discharge orders, the doctor will let you get dressed and leave, assisted by a friend or relative, as it is unsafe to drive after receiving the IV medication. You will likely be given instructions on diet following the endoscopic procedure that may include a liquid diet for a day or longer or specifications that you chew your food well. In the next few days, the previously mentioned side effects from surgery may crop up. Be sure to call the doctor with any of the changes.

The fundoplication surgery is another ball game altogether since an overnight stay is likely to be ordered and the prep is a little more involved. Because of this, you will not be able to simply waltz into the hospital on the day of the procedure. Instead, your preparation for surgery will begin at home.

Before you leave for the hospital, request a list of foods that you will be able to have following surgery and then stock up your pantry. Ask for any prescriptions that you may need following surgery so they can be filled ahead of time. This eliminates any such steps you will feel less like doing when you are in pain or not quite recovered following the procedure.

In packing for the hospital, keep things light. Don't bring any valuables but do bring the things that make you feel comfortable at home. Your favorite slippers (preferably with a nonskid sole), a nightshirt that buttons up the front (to make changing with an IV bag that much easier and to avoid raising the hands over the head following the procedure) or similar loose clothing may be better than anything that the hospital can provide. You may also want to pack your pillow and your toiletries, as the hospital offerings always seem to fall a little short in this category. Soft, spongy earplugs, available in most drugstores or in target ranges, are usually quite cheap and will help to block out the evening noise and the roommate's snores.

Some doctors and hospitals require that the bowel prep be done beforehand at home while others will administer it right as you arrive in your room after registration. In any case, it helps to be prepared ahead of time. The doctor will prescribe one of several bowel cleansing preparations to be taken. Some are worse than others but all do the same thing: strip everything from the walls of your digestive tract and force it through as quickly as possible. In addition to the prep, be sure that you have soft toilet paper (one preferred brand is Kleenex Cottonelle with aloe and vitamin E), petroleum jelly, plenty of hemorrhoid cream, and a good supply of reading material with you. Use the petroleum jelly first to lubricate the anus. This will help to protect the sensitive tissues there from being burned by any quickly exiting caustic material such as unabsorbed digestive enzymes. After quickly drinking the liquid or swallowing the pills, do not stray too far from the bathroom, as you will soon have to go like you have never had to go before. As you are emptying out, continue to wipe and flush often, following up with a generous portion of the cream applied to the anus at the end of the event. You may feel cold or shaky after the bowel cleanse, a natural reaction to depletion of electrolytes, or your muscles may ache. If this is the case, a warm bath will do the trick.

Prior to surgery and after changing into the surgical gown, you will have an IV line inserted. You can request a sedative at this time if you are nervous (and who isn't?). An anesthesiologist will likely discuss what will be administered to you and assure you that your condition will be monitored throughout the surgery. The surgeon will also likely discuss the procedure that is to be performed and answer any questions you might have. The support personnel may seem like they are asking a lot of questions regarding your procedure, as if they are verifying that you are who you say you are and that you are having done what you say you are having done. Don't worry. They are doing just that. No one likes to go in to have the laparoscopic Nissen fundoplication only to wake up without a gallbladder. The staff is just making sure that this doesn't happen.

Following surgery, you will be wheeled into the recovery room. You may feel a little nauseous and experience a sore throat and a parched mouth. This is common in GI surgeries. You may have a nasogastric tube inserted to relieve pressure in the stomach, a catheter inserted to collect urine, and an oxygen tube resting in the space between your upper lip and your nose. In time, the tubes will be removed.

You may not feel like leaving your bed following surgery but try anyway. Moving your body helps your bowels to move more quickly again, even if you haven't eaten anything. And once your bowels begin to move, you will begin to eat again and will likely be discharged more quickly. Your goal at first should not be to be doing laps around the nursing station because you don't want to overdo it. Instead, just try making it to the bathroom and back for the first time, setting a further goal each time you get out of bed. Also, you may be asked to suck on a strange plastic contraption, the colorful plastic balls in which rise as you do so. This is an incentive spirometer and it helps you to maintain proper lung function following surgery. Humor them and do it; you'll be better off for it.

When you return home, take it easy and be sure to follow the doctor's discharge notes. Rely on others to help out with chores and driving duties until you are well enough to do so. Unless you are a total wretch, they are likely looking for an opportunity to help you during your time of need.

Diet tips for the weeks following surgery and endoscopic procedures

IMMEDIATELY FOLLOWING THE endoscopic procedures, your doctor may prescribe, in addition to a pain killer, a diet for you to follow. The diet usually consists of at least one meal that is clear liquids and moves up through soft foods to a regular diet in less than a week. Usually not anything that would be served in a five-star setting, the diet is intended to allow the area around the LES to continue healing with the least amount of strain. To assure the best results possible, it is important to follow the diet to the letter.

For those recovering from the fundoplication surgery, a return to eating normally may take a little while longer as the body adjusts to having a tighter LES and a possibly newly elongated esophagus.

When Robin was recovering from his laparoscopic Nissen fundoplication procedure in the hospital, his first tray of food was topped off with a can of Coca-Cola. "Someone had made a mistake. The last thing a fresh fundo patient needs is anything carbonated," he said.

In the following days and weeks, he kept his diet to mostly soft foods such as puddings, soft or mashed vegetables, fried or soft-boiled eggs, applesauce, pureed soups, and yogurt as well as noncarbonated beverages such as water, fruit juices, tea, and milkshakes. He stayed away from carbonated beverages due to the burping factor, alcohol because of its possible interaction with pain medication, gassy vegetables (cauliflower, cabbage, broccoli, and beans) for obvious reasons, and meat and bread, as they tended to "hang" in his esophagus. Gradually in the month after his surgery, he was able to add soft fruits and vegetables such as avocado, ripe melon, peaches, and tomatoes as well as broiled fish and pasta. Red meat was cautiously added and well chewed in the next month and, with the exception of bread, he was able to return to a normal diet during that time. Bread continues to give him trouble on occasion, something he remedies by drinking warm water to counteract the problem with sticking.

"Within six to eight weeks after surgery, I was eating a normal diet including red meat—small bites chewed very well. Bread continued to give me troubles for another month or so. Even then, for the next three or four months I would occasionally have bread hang in my esophagus," Robin said. "Today, more than thirteen months postfundo, there isn't anything I can't eat, although I must say I am far more conscious of eating a well-balanced diet."

Additionally, some individuals find that they can experience nausea or spasms due to the gas-bloat syndrome. There are antispasmodic medications such as Levsin, Bentyl, or Levbid that can help with the spasms but be forewarned that they are also anticholinergic and can slow the movements of your intestines. There are antinausea medications such as Compazine that can ease that symptom as well.

QUESTIONS FOR THE PHYSICIAN

MAYBE YOU have tried everything—all medications and lifestyle modifications—and nothing works. Perhaps you just can't imagine taking medication day after day into eternity. Or you are just one of those unlucky souls who has an extraesophageal condition that medication just can't surmount.

Whatever the case, you are now in the surgeon's office, ready to start your first consultation for surgery. What happens in the next few minutes can change the outcome of your surgery so it is important to be prepared with all of the questions you have ahead of time. Sue Ann knows what that is like. Before she went through a laparoscopic Nissen fundoplication to ease her symptoms of GERD, she prepared for the event by drawing up a five-page, typewritten list of questions to ask the surgeon.

Below is a list of suggested questions for the surgeon or physician, some

continued

from Sue Ann's original list and others from personal surgical experience. Feel free to extract what you would like to ask and add a few of your own. At the time you meet the physician and ask these questions, it helps to have them printed out. As a courtesy, you might also offer the physician his or her own copy so he or she can follow along. Also, be sure to bring other paper and a writing instrument to record his or her answers, as you will likely forget some of what is said.

1. How much experience do you have with the antireflux surgical or endoscopic procedures? Can you tell me how long you have been doing it, how many procedures you have done, and where you learned it?
2. How many patients are you currently seeing who have either just had the surgery or procedure or are contemplating having it?
3. How would you work with the other doctors who are treating me?
4. What tests do you plan to perform on me prior to the surgery or endoscopic procedure? Why?
5. For surgery, what techniques do you favor? Why? Do you do more open surgery or laparotomy?
6. What is the complication rate you have experienced? What kind of complications have you encountered? What is your fatality rate? What happened in those circumstances?
7. What can I expect regarding the surgical or endoscopic experience on the day of the event? How long does the procedure take?
8. What can I expect of my recovery? When will I be mobile again? What kind of special diet will I have to follow and for how long? Will I be able to sleep on a level bed again? Will I still have to take acid-reducing medication?
9. Who will be in the operating room or endoscopic suite with you? (This is a good question to ask if the facility is a teaching hospital and a student may partake in the procedure). Will you be doing all of the work?
10. What types of pain management techniques do you employ?
11. If I have an emergency following the procedure, what is the protocol I should follow to get in touch with you? Do you work with other doctors with similar experience who would be able to handle the call if you were not available? Under what circumstances should I call you?
12. How do you feel about alternative medicine and treatments?

One final note: Do not feel compelled to go only to the surgeon to whom you are referred. If you do not click with this person or do not feel completely confident with his or her abilities, find another physician to take your case.

6

ALTERNATIVE TREATMENTS

Before there were MDs and DOs, before there were certified medical schools and specialties, before the endoscope and even the stethoscope, there was still medicine. There were tribal medicine men on this continent and others who acted as the local expert on medical issues; there were women who practiced female medicine in their villages, coaching women through their pregnancies and childbirths. These early medical professionals performed rituals to chase away demons that were assumed to cause conditions or danced to entice better spirits to cure an individual. They also used nature to provide relief for a myriad of conditions, including heartburn.

While the dances and the rituals have mostly fallen by the wayside, some of the early treatments for GERD remain today and are becoming increasingly relied upon by a public more interested in natural therapies to complement their more traditional medicine. These time-tested herbal therapies are sold in common pharmacies while ancient pain and stress reduction techniques are taught in strip malls and community gymnasiums across the country. According to the National Health and Nutrition Examination Survey, 42 percent of Americans spent $27 billion on complementary and alternative medicine, including many people who forked over cash in search of a natural way of dealing with their raging reflux. And the governmentally supported, pro-Western medicine mentality that has held for centuries is slowly giving way to some of the more Eastern-based practices such as tai chi and yoga as a new division of the National Institutes of Health, the National Center for Complementary and Alternative Medicine, was opened recently. Its goal is to apply Western-based study techniques such as double-blind, placebo controlled studies to such practices as ayurveda and guided imagery.

Like medications, the herbs and natural supplements usually have some intended action in the body, as you will discover below; some, for example, act as anti-inflammatory agents on a scorched esophageal mucosa while others are intended to soothe a nauseous tummy. Unlike medications, however, their dosage and strength can vary from manufacturer to manufacturer, from batch to batch, from bottle to bottle. As a result, your benefits may also vary.

While it may seem that nearly everyone is seeking some sort of natural therapy or supplement, it is important to realize that it should be done with the knowledge of your physician. Some herbs, such as St. John's wort, have been shown in clinical studies to interact with antidepressant medication, for example, and others can decrease the effectiveness of certain drugs taken for cardiovascular disease. Because of the possibility of herb-drug interaction, it is important to discuss all natural therapies or supplements you are thinking of taking with your doctor before you even buy them. Also, you may want to consult a trusted herbalist or naturopathic specialist to find the proper usage of the herbs.

Herbs that may help

BELOW ARE DIFFERENT herbs and supplements that may provide relief of certain GERD symptoms:

■ *Aloe vera juice.* Three millennia ago, the ancient Egyptians used this tropical and subtropical pointy plant to soothe burns and help heal cuts, and hundreds of other societies have used it for the same reasons since then. No one is really sure why it works, since the gel inside the fat leaves is about 96 percent water, but it is believed that naturally occurring pectin in the leaves stimulates a growth hormone and prompts new cell formation. Whatever the case, some individuals with GERD mix a gel concentrate with juice or tea and drink it to soothe a case of esophagitis. Aside from the unpleasant taste, the gel may also have a laxative effect so it is wise to use it with caution, especially with medications that can lower potassium, such as digoxin or diuretics. It can also interfere with some diabetes medications.

- *Barley grass*. Usually a concoction made from juice extracted from young barley grass, this substance is rich in amino acids and in chlorophyll. It has natural anti-inflammatory properties.

- *Chamomile and fennel seed teas*. Given to babies in a weak tea to settle a case of colic, these folk remedies, best prepared in the tea form, are soothing to the gastrointestinal system in that they reduce gas and cramping. Beware, however: some individuals find that they are sensitive to these properties and experience a *worsening* of their symptoms as the LES also relaxes. Be careful if you take sedatives or blood thinners since the herbs can magnify those effects.

- *Charcoal*. If gas is the issue that keeps a case of reflux bubbling up, one commonly used supplement that some individuals turn to is activated charcoal (Charcocaps). Usually, the dose is two to four capsules taken before mealtime and an hour following a meal. Be warned, however, that this will change the color of the stool to black and may mask any bleeding of the intestines as a result.

- *Cilantro and coriander seeds*. Parts of the same plant, these two items have been prescribed by midwives for millennia to quell cases of pregnancy-related nausea. Women then would chew on the cilantro leaves or the coriander seeds or would make a tea with either. Both cilantro and coriander seeds can be found in the aisles of any well-stocked grocery store.

- *Ginger*. That little lump of pink stuff served next to your sushi does more than simply perk up the plate and cleanse your palate. In fact, it is there because it is seen as a digestive aid in Asian culture. Another mid-wife secret, this root has been used for four thousand years in a number of cultures to settle cases of pregnancy-related nausea. In GERD, individuals have been known to make a juice out of the root, to chew on slices of the root, to eat crystallized particles made of the root, or to swallow capsules or teas containing bits of the root.

- *Licorice root*. Long a staple of Chinese medicine, licorice has been used in a variety of applications for a number of conditions. In GERD, licorice is used by some herbalists as an anti-inflammatory in those with esophagitis; it must mix with saliva so a tea or a chewable tablet works the best, as opposed to a capsule that would bypass the problem. Because licorice can cause an increase in blood pressure in certain individuals, some people prefer to take DGL, or deglycyrrhizin licorice, which removes the potential culprit, glycyrrhizin.

- *Linden.* Like the slippery elm, this is a derivative of a tree and is also a type of soothing mucilage. Used in old European cultures, the flowers of the tree are generally dried and used to brew a tea or pressed to extract the essence. People with reflux sometimes use linden to soothe a case of esophagitis and as an anti-spasmodic in a spastic esophagus.

- *Marshmallow.* Not to be confused with the sticky staple ingredient of Moon Pies and S'mores, this plant has been used for centuries by Arabic cultures as a type of anti-inflammatory salve. The plant's root and leaves contain soothing mucilage that is often used in conjunction with chamomile in a tea or in an extract for an inflamed esophagus in GERD.

- *Meadowsweet.* With properties that are consistent with salicylic acid (aspirin), one might think that this herb is simply a pain reliever. However, teas and extracts made from the flowers of the plant have also been found to have anti-inflammatory and antacid qualities, making this herb a choice for some people with symptomatic GERD.

- *Slippery elm bark.* This gruel or powder, mixed with water and consumed, was made from bark that was stripped from the trees and used by early American pioneers as food and as medicine for upset stomachs. Known as mucilage, it coats the esophagus and soothes a case of esophagitis. It is also sold in large capsules but these may not have the desired effect as the benefit comes from the direct contact of the elm bark on the mucosa and the capsules don't open until after they pass through the esophagus.

HERBS THAT CAN HURT

NOT ALL HERBS and supplements that are used for general gastrointestinal distress will be beneficial for individuals with GERD; in fact, some may actually cause a worsening of symptoms.

- *Peppermint and spearmint.* These two herbs are tasty in gums and teas or when eaten raw. They are also commonly used to quiet a spastic colon or ease a belly distended from too much eating. But in people with GERD, they can relax the one thing that may actually need to be more taut: the LES. Because of this effect, many doctors advise patients to avoid after-dinner mints and other items containing mint.

■ ■ ■

Digestive enzymes

OUR BODIES SECRETE enzymes to speed up the chemical processes in a variety of situations, with digestion being one such incidence that is repeated several times daily. In the stomach, food and beverages containing protein are greeted with pepsin, which, along with mucus, hydrochloric acid, and the grinding motion of the stomach muscles, helps to make the initial chunks of food into more of a liquid stew that empties into the small intestine where it is more easily absorbed. The pancreas then dribbles into the duodenum lipase to break down fats and amylase to break down starch. Other digestive enzymes work to further break down certain sugars throughout the small intestine; for example, the milk sugar lactose is degraded by the digestive enzyme lactase in the small and large intestine. All of this metabolic action is essential to allow the body to properly absorb the specific nutrients.

The vast majority of people in the world secrete enough such enzymes that supplementation is unnecessary. However, some people lack enough of a certain enzyme or enzymes and must supplement their diets with synthetically produced enzymes. For example, those with cystic fibrosis take supplements to help digest foods while those with lactose intolerance may take a pill to allow them to consume ice cream or milk without a wicked case of gas that would follow if they didn't. Many people with pancreatic diseases such as pancreatic cancer must take enzymes as the pancreas is impaired; those with gastroparesis may have to take supplemental enzymes as well.

Currently, there are no well-controlled studies to support a theory that supplementing with digestive enzymes would improve symptoms of reflux because it would aid in digestion, thus making things move along more quickly through the stomach. Many of the supplemental enzymes are not acid-resistant and must be protected in some fashion to keep them from releasing in the stomach; once in the intestines, the enzymes are released and do their work.

Pain and stress reduction techniques

FOR SOME INDIVIDUALS, pain is inherent with GERD. They experience pain when they swallow, shortly after a meal, while sleeping, or while exercising. While some relief can come in a bottle, it can also come from various activities, both mental and physical, various studies show.

■　■　■

FIVE WAYS TO REDUCE PAIN AND STRESS

1. Meditation or guided imagery
2. Massage
3. Acupressure, acupuncture, or reflexology
4. Biofeedback
5. Yoga or tai chi

Additionally, stress has been shown to exacerbate or initiate a number of illnesses, GERD included. When people are under stress, they don't sleep as well or eat as well and their immune systems take a dive, making them susceptible to a number of illnesses or worsening the ones they already have. The stress can come from having the illness or can be related to everyday situations we encounter, such as relationship issues and work problems. Studies show that people with health problems associated with any form of stress can see a reduction in symptoms if the afflicted person employs some form of regular stress reduction technique such as meditation or exercise.

So it makes sense, then, that a person would feel better if he or she were able to reduce the amount of both pain and stress in their lives. Still, anyone who is embarking on an exercise program or any of the below mentioned techniques—however gentle they may seem—would be wise to consult a physician first.

- *Meditation and guided imagery.* One of the easiest ways of diverting the mind from pain and stress is to literally divert the mind. Usually, this type of mental exercise is performed in a soothing room environment, either on a comfortable piece of furniture or in a comfortable position on the floor, with little or no distractions present. The individual then closes his or her eyes, gradually and progressively allowing various muscle groups to go slack while focusing on breathing. Imagery involves the same relaxation techniques but adds the mind's ability to travel to a relaxing and pleasing place. Both techniques have been documented to slow heart rate, reduce blood pressure, decrease pain perception, and release tension.
- *Massage.* The healing sense of touch is found in massage, another way of relaxing the body without putting forth too much effort. Studies have shown that massage— from Reiki to shiatsu, from a sports massage to a pedicure, and everything in

between—not only releases stress and tension from muscles while decreasing pain perception but also provides a mental benefit brought about by the simple act of human touch.

■ *Acupressure, acupuncture, and reflexology.* These are also fairly docile ways of reducing stress, decreasing pain, and reducing nausea. Acupressure and acupuncture are based on the Chinese belief that energy flows throughout the body in patterns and that when these patterns are disrupted, pain exists. Through acupuncture, thin needles are inserted fairly painlessly into pressure points known as meridians to restore a positive flow and reduce pain. In acupressure, no needles are used but instead the practitioner places pressure on the meridians for a certain amount of time to achieve the same results. Recent studies have found that these benefits can be scientifically proven; as a result, many hospitals offer the services of an acupressurist or an acupuncturist as adjunctive therapy to postsurgical patients. In GERD patients, some people find relief from pain and nausea due to a pressure point that is located below the sternum and above the navel. In reflexology, the pressure points are found most commonly in the sole of the foot, less commonly in the hands or ear lobes. For GERD pain, the spot that spells relief is located south of the major pad on the big toe.

■ *Biofeedback.* This is a fairly new and controversial approach to medicine. The theory behind it is that the body can be trained to recognize involuntary changes in the body and correct them before an adverse event occurs. To achieve this, electrodes are placed on the body and record such things as heart rate, body temperature, blood pressure, and involuntary muscle contractions or relaxations; in GERD, the relaxation of the LES is tracked. Through several sessions, the patient is trained to recognize these changes and to manipulate these changes in a positive manner to avoid an undesirable result. Although a cloud of controversy has followed the practice of biofeedback, some people with GERD swear by it.

■ *Yoga and tai chi.* Popular as never before, yoga and tai chi have become healthy exercise alternatives as well as wonderfully relaxing ways to relieve stress. Numerous studies have shown that people who regularly practice yoga and tai chi have been able to slow their heart rate and reduce their blood pressure. While some forms of yoga can really work up a sweat during an arduous workout, others are more meditative and gentle, allowing for various flexibilities and different levels of skill; tai chi combines more gentle movements and is an excellent alternative for those whose motion is restricted. For those about to try their first downward facing dog pose or taking in that first tai chi class, it is wise to abstain from eating for at least two to four hours beforehand to allow for digestion. Also, you may want to discuss your specific health issue with the yoga practitioner or the tai chi leader prior to a class and ask if all of the poses and movements will be appropriate for you to perform.

7

REFLUX IN PREGNANCY, CHILDHOOD, AND SENIOR ADULTHOOD

IF YOU BELIEVED the ads on television or in magazines, it would appear that everyone who had reflux was a) an adult between the ages of forty and fifty, b) gluttonous (i.e., "I can't believe I ate the whole thing"), and c) male.

But that is not the case. What is glaringly missing in those very ads are the individuals who have reflux and are a) below the age of sixteen, b) above the age of sixty-five, and c) pregnant. These patients can be just as miserable—if not more miserable—than the more typical reflux patient who might fit that advertising profile. These subgroups of reflux patients have special needs and concerns that the more traditional and courted patient body with reflux do not have. Included in these interests are the effects of medication with regard to their age or condition, special concerns regarding surgical options and outcomes, as well as heightened attention to nutritional needs when food does not stay down or is avoided because it is associated with pain. For these reasons, pregnant women, children, and the elderly are and should be treated differently.

■　■　■

Reflux in Pregnancy

PREGNANCY CAN BE a wonderful time in a woman's life, filled with expectation and promise as the body blooms before one's very eyes. Expectant mothers are often pictured with a hand on the enlarged tummy, a head full of glossy hair, and bright, sparkling eyes. But the reality often can be much, much different. Hope and joy aside, pregnancy can be downright hellish, filled with bad hair days and swollen limbs. And that doesn't even begin to touch the increased risk and intensity of reflux that commonly joins a resurgence of acne and the appearance of stretch marks as the overlooked realities of this otherwise blessed time.

Studies regarding the incidence rates of reflux during pregnancy find varying rates, ranging from one-quarter of all pregnant women having daily symptoms from the get go to 72 percent experiencing some level of heartburn severity in the third trimester. What some of the findings seem to have in common is that there is an increase in the number of women who have daily heartburn the further into gestation the pregnancy progresses.

No one is exactly sure why this phenomenon occurs but there are plenty of theories, all of which are plausible. For one, the shifting levels of hormones during pregnancy, particularly progesterone and estrogen, can cause changes in the way the GI tract operates. As an example, progesterone in higher levels in the pregnant body causes the GI tract to relax, not a good thing for the LES. Also, progesterone, paired with the constipating effect of the iron-rich prenatal vitamins prescribed during pregnancy, can lead to decreased bowel motility and an increase in time that food takes to leave the stomach, known factors for a rip-roaring case of acid reflux.

Another possible reason for the increase in heartburn among pregnant women can be found in the logistics of carrying a growing fetus inside the body. As the fetus develops from a tiny, nearly weightless speck to that of a multi-pound, full-sized being, the body must adjust to accommodate sharing the living space, so to speak. In many ways, it is like moving a second person into a one-person studio apartment. Just as you would have to move some furniture around to adjust to the extra resident, the female body has to slightly displace some organs in the normal anatomy to accommodate the fetus. As the fetus grows, it presses the intestines upward, placing greater pressure on the stomach. That force alone can cause the LES to open and stomach contents to reflux into the esophagus. Aside from the constant pressure of the growing fetus, additional, transient jabs can occur when the fetus kicks or moves upward sharply.

Still another potential reason for the increase in heartburn during pregnancy can be attributed to some habits and lifestyle choices that pregnant women are known to make. For example, some pregnant women continue to wear their nonmaternity clothing as long as possible, perhaps in denial that their body is actually growing. Also, some fashionistas feel the need to embrace the trends of tighter maternity clothing, despite the extra pressure it might make on their growing abdomen. The tight clothing places external pressure on the stomach, possibly foreshadowing a reflux event. Other women find that their hunger is nearly impossible to quench and give in to eating large meals or at inconvenient times, such as right before bedtime or in the middle of the night. Still others find that they crave certain foods during certain points in their pregnancy, foods that can cause reflux in a relatively healthy, nonpregnant person; therefore, eating a jar of pickles in one sitting, drinking a gallon of tomato juice in a three-day period, or constantly nibbling on chocolate may not be the best idea, no matter how tasty it sounds at the time. Finally, some women are relegated to bed rest due to complications in their pregnancy. Because of this, their movement is limited and their ability to remain upright may be compromised, leading to heartburn.

For diagnostic purposes, many doctors prefer to treat the symptoms without subjecting the pregnant patient to the testing they would normally undergo if they were not pregnant. This is in part due to the fact that so many women experience such digestive problems during pregnancy but also because some of the tests, especially those involving the radiation of Xrays or the sedation of the patient, could have negative effects on the fetus. If endoscopy is necessary due to such factors as bleeding or weight loss, some doctors prefer to delay it until after the first trimester, using conscious sedation that is safe for pregnant women.

For the most part, doctors try first to alleviate symptoms of pregnancy-related heartburn by suggesting some lifestyle modifications, opting for medication when these changes fail. Eating smaller but more frequent meals, avoiding foods and beverages that trigger heartburn, drinking more water, and wearing maternity clothing with more forgiving waistlines can help achieve results in some people with daytime heartburn.

For nighttime attacks, eliminating bedtime snacks and middle of the night food orgies can go a long way to preventing heartburn. Changing your sleeping position can also make a dent in the severity and frequency of attacks. Many obstetricians ask that their pregnant patients lie on their left side when they sleep to reduce pressure on certain arteries that supply blood to the legs and to reduce pressure on the liver, located on the right side in the upper abdomen; at the same time, many gastroenterologists suggest that heartburn patients can reduce nighttime occurrences by elevating the head and upper torso to allow gravity to keep stomach contents from rising into the esophagus. To achieve both, using lots of extra pillows is key. It helps to sleep with a pillow between the knees and a pillow to prop the small of the back in place as well as extra pillows or a wedge to elevate the head and upper torso. If this seems like a lot to go through for a good night's sleep, it is, but it increases the chances of snagging some uninterrupted ZZZs before the baby comes, causing further sleep deprivation.

When lifestyle modifications are not successful in controlling acid reflux, doctors might suggest combining the lifestyle modifications with some over-the-counter or prescription medications. However, great caution is exercised in doing so, as medications are known to pass through the placenta to the forming embryo or fetus.

When the embryonic or fetal exposure to medication occurs and what type of medication is given can determine whether there will be an effect on the embryo or fetus and how mild or severe the damage will be. If there is exposure to medication in the first two weeks following conception, the embryo will either dissolve or fix the damage and continue to develop. The next key stage continues through the end of the first trimester when exposure to harmful substances can impair the growth of internal organs and other features, leading to the loss of the pregnancy. However, this is just one of many reasons that pregnancies are lost during this stage. Harmful substances continue to pose a risk for the developing fetus for the rest of the pregnancy as the brain develops; exposure to these substances and certain medications can result in behavioral or developmental issues in the years to come. Again, even in babies born to the healthiest of patients who are taking no medications or exposed to no harmful substances, there is still a 3 to 5 percent risk of congenital abnormalities or birth defects.

UNDERSTANDING FDA DRUG RANKINGS FOR PREGNANCY

IT IS important to understand how the medications for reflux are categorized and what risks they pose to the mother and the fetus. The Food and Drug Administration (FDA), a governmental agency charged with the task of approving medications for use by the American public, has created an alphabet-based ranking system for drugs used in pregnancies.

- The first category, A, is for drugs that have been proven in adequate studies of pregnant women not to harm to the fetus. There are very few drugs in this category across the board.

continued

- Category B drugs are defined as those for which animal studies show no risk to the fetus, but there are as yet no adequate or well controlled studies regarding pregnant women; additionally, drugs in this category may have shown a negative effect on animal fetuses but adequate, well-controlled studies in pregnant women have not shown the same outcome. This is a fairly wide category.
- Category C drugs have no adequate, well-controlled studies involving pregnant women and either have had no animal studies to prove or disprove risk to fetal development or the studies have shown a negative effect on the animal fetal development.
- Category D drugs have been documented in adequate, well-controlled studies to potentially cause harm to the fetus; these drugs can still be used in certain patients when the benefits outweigh the risk.
- Category X drugs have been shown in studies definitively to cause abortive effects on the pregnancy or deformities in the fetus. These drugs should not be used under any circumstance during pregnancy.

It is important to note that none of the medications used in the treatment of reflux fall into categories A, D, or X. Additionally, many new drugs fall into category C and may be moved to other categories as research proves whether they are safe to use in pregnancy or not. At the same time, some drugs that are initially listed as category B drugs may move to category C if negative case reports are filed after the drugs are marketed.

As we have already seen, there is room in the treatment of acid reflux disease for doctors to develop their own approaches to treatment. For example, some physicians skip over the antacids, normally seen as a first line of defense in GERD. This is because the antacids, while immediately controlling the problem, have possible side effects that could potentially cause problems for the pregnant woman. For one, antacids with aluminum salts are great because there is no acid rebound in them like some containing calcium, but they carry with them the unfortunate side effect of potentially intensifying constipation normally experienced during pregnancy, a side effect that can aid in the formation of painful hemorrhoids. Those with sodium bicarbonate can cause water retention and metabolic alkalosis, a term that is used to describe a condition in which a shift occurs between acid and alkalinity in the body, which can lead to the loss of potassium. Other magnesium-containing antacids can offset labor in some individuals; for example, magnesium sulfate often is used to stop preterm labor in some women. But other doctors find that taking an occasional antacid, such as one combined with alginic acid, works well for temporary heartburn relief.

All of the most commonly prescribed H$_2$ RAs are category B medications and are considered safe to take during pregnancy, at the over-the-counter dosage level or the prescription level. In paperwork filed with the FDA, Tagamet (cimetidine), Zantac (ranitidine hydrochloride), Axid (nizatidine), and Mylanta and Pepcid (both containing famotidine) are all listed as category B medications. Only one, Pepcid, listed any problems in animal control studies; in that instance, some rabbits that were given what would be greater than 250 times the normal human dosage were found to decrease their food intake and experience spontaneous abortion. However, there are no adequate or well-controlled tests on pregnant women. Nizatidine is somewhat controversial in that some animal studies have shown deleterious effects to the fetus such as low fetal weight and spontaneous abortions.

Of the PPIs, most of the most commonly prescribed drugs—(esomeprazole) Nexium, (rabeprazole) AcipHex, (lansoprazole) Prevacid, and (pantoprazole) Protonix —are category B drugs. In pregnant rabbits that took anywhere from 17 to 172 times the human dosage of (omeprazole) Prilosec, scientists found that there were dose-related increases in problems with pregnancies such as fetal resorption and death of the embryo; pregnant rats and their forthcoming offspring suffered dose-related complications as well. In humans, there have been reports of congenital abnormalities in the babies born to mothers who took omeprazole during their pregnancy. Because of these reports, the drug is considered a category C drug. Because Nexium is a close relative of Prilosec, some doctors use caution in prescribing this drug as well.

As for other medications that are often used in conjunction with GERD drugs, it is a mixed bag. Sucralfate, the medication that is used by few doctors to increase mucosal resistance to acid, is a category B drug because it is generally not systemically absorbed. Metoclopramide, the side-effect-ridden prokinetic agent, is a category B drug, but its side effects of anxiety and insomnia may not exactly endear it to the pregnant woman.

The bad news about taking these medications is that all of these drugs can be excreted in human milk and could potentially cause an adverse reaction in a nursing infant, such as delayed weight gain. Because of this, it is important to consult a physician about taking the medication after the birth and during lactation. The good news is that reflux generally resolves itself in the days, weeks, and months following birth as weight is lost and hormone levels return to normal, leaving little need for medication in most women.

Reflux in childhood

EVERY BABY SPITS up. And, sometimes, it is even a little cute.

But when it happens often, when it is accompanied by fits of screaming, projectile vomiting, drops of blood in the spit up, arching of the back, and general unpleasantness associated with eating and sleeping, it could be a classic case of childhood GERD. Although many infantile cases of reflux correct themselves within two years of birth, some children can continue to experience these symptoms for years, or develop others such as GERD-related asthma and other lung complications, chronic ear infections, low weight, esophagitis, strictures, and Barrett's esophagus. In particular, many children whose neurological function is impaired may suffer from any of these symptoms continually.

The symptoms of reflux in children are the same as in adults but certain symptoms, such as vomiting and aspiration of the reflux resulting in asthma or chronic lung infections, are more common in children, while other common adult symptoms, such as chest pain, are less common in children. There are also certain symptoms in children, such as a peculiar arching of the neck as well as sinus and ear infections, that are not widely present in adults. Other symptoms shared by these different age groups include sore throats with or without esophagitis, pain that wakes them in the middle of the night, difficulty swallowing, refusal of food to the point of weight loss (or, in the case of very young children, poor growth or inadequate weight gain), sleep apnea, and acid-related tooth enamel damage.

The diagnosis of reflux in children is also more complicated than it is in adults. Obviously, this may be due to the fact that small children may not be able to articulate their pain; in other words, a baby will not be able to say that the spitting up is hurting his or her throat and that is why he or she doesn't want to eat. At the same time, older children who have always had these symptoms since birth may think that everyone must share these symptoms and therefore see their condition as abnormal and *not* shared by other children their age. These children, for example, may think it is normal to vomit every now and then after eating and not report these incidents as they occur.

To complicate matters more, often the signs and symptoms of reflux are shared by other conditions. Common symptoms suffered by infants with reflux include vomiting, chronic spitting up, food refusal, and problems with swallowing. However, those same symptoms are shared by other conditions including food allergies, metabolic dysfunction, and structural abnormalities such as esophageal atresia, a condition in which the esophagus is incompletely formed and possibly disconnected from the stomach. Even something as simple as an infant accidentally sticking its fingers or hand too far in the throat and initiating a gag reflex can cause vomiting. In older children and adolescents, vomiting and food refusal can be caused by inflammatory bowel diseases such as Crohn's disease; by bowel obstructions caused by noninflammatory, mechanical conditions such as intussusception, a circumstance caused by the telescoping of the intestines on themselves; by food allergies; or, in the case of postpubescent adolescent girls, pregnancy.

Doctors employ the same tests in children to diagnose reflux and rule out other conditions as they do in adults. Barium Xrays are often used to rule out any congenital malformations or strictures. Esophagogastroduodenoscopy, performed with pediatric downsized endoscopes, will allow the doctor to see any pathological changes to the mucosa while also giving him or her access to biopsies of these areas. The 24-hour ambulatory pH monitoring may also be conducted in cases where esophagitis is not present. Esophageal manometry, albeit with smaller equipment, can be done to detect normal or abnormal motility in the esophagus. Scintigraphy can also show if a child is experiencing gastric motility issues; in the case of infants who are not yet consuming solid foods, their formula is often laced with radiolabeled substances to facilitate the viewing of its movement.

The causes or prompts of infantile or childhood reflux are, in many cases, different than those adults experience. Wearing tight clothing or smoking are two things that children don't often do, nor do they typically have a spicy diet or drink alcohol. Instead, infants usually experience transient relaxation of the LES that may be attributable to an undeveloped neurological response. As their voluntary and involuntary reflexes mature during the first year and beyond, most of the infants with reflux symptoms see a decline in or disappearance of symptoms by the time they celebrate their second birthday. However, a small number of children, some with neurological development issues and others who are otherwise healthy, will continue to struggle with the signs and symptoms of reflux beyond that time frame.

Treatment options for children are not as wide or encompassing as they are for adults, partly because parents aren't usually as willing to submit their children as test subjects for medication-approval purposes. Usually, a pediatric gastroenterologist or the child's pediatrician first will suggest lifestyle modifications, largely related to eating and sleeping, in order to treat the condition. One change parents can make to ease the symptoms of their child is to make sure that the child is held vertically during and after mealtime, allowing gravity to keep the stomach's contents from splashing back into the esophagus; not allowing eating prior to nap or bedtime is also helpful. Another lifestyle alteration is to add heft in the form of oat or rice infant cereal to the child's meals, using weight to diminish the chance of stomach contents easily splashing into the esophagus.

One somewhat controversial lifestyle modification that some doctors suggest to the parents of the infant patients is to place the child on its stomach while sleeping. In the past few years, this position has been linked to sudden infant death syndrome (SIDS), a condition that several studies suggest is rectified if the child is placed on its back during sleep. But doing so, some doctors argue, places the junction of the stomach and the esophagus below the fluid line, allowing the reflux to take place. Doctors also say that SIDS is more likely related to placing fluffy bedding in the crib where the child can suffocate; placing a child on its stomach on a tight bed sheet should cause no greater risk, they say. This position then allows gravity to keep the stomach contents away from the LES, lessening the chance of reflux. The American Academy of Pediatrics Task Force on Infant Positioning and SIDS backs up these exceptions by issuing recommendations that include the following statement: "The current recommendation is for healthy infants only. The pediatrician should consider the relative risks and benefits. Gastroesophageal reflux and certain upper airway anomalies that predispose to airway obstruction and perhaps some other illnesses may be indications for a prone sleeping position." Because this issue remains controversial, it is important for parents to discuss sleeping position with the child's doctor.

Another sleep modification a parent can make to ease symptoms is to place the child's crib on books or a support to raise the head of the crib or bed. By doing so, gravity again is allowed to work in reducing the chance of refluxed stomach contents. This technique is often used with children who have sinus infections or colds so as to aid the mucus discharge in emptying down the back of the child's throat. There are two areas of concern: having the crib slide off the supports and having the child slide down the mattress. The first can be remedied with certain safety products designed to raise the head of the bed without raising the bed entirely. One is the Safe Lift Crib Wedge by Dex Baby Products, a covered, firm foam wedge that is inserted above the mattress and beneath the sheets. Another option is crib or bed risers, cone-shaped blocks of durable plastic with impressions in the tops in which to place the crib legs; hardware can be used to secure the furniture legs to certain risers. Placing the child in a terry-cloth sleeper on a combed cotton or flannel crib sheet may rectify the second issue, as the friction between the two fabrics can slow the slide. Another way of solving the problem is to use a product called the Tucker Sling, a combination of a sheet that fits over the top portion of the mattress and a seat that secures over the infant's clothing that virtually assures no twisting, turning, or sliding of the child down the mattress.

A third sleep modification addresses the issue of sleep apnea, a condition that has been found to be higher in children with reflux. Since the episodes of this can be life threatening, some children are placed on an apnea monitor, a small device that is strapped on a child's chest and sounds an alarm when breathing stops for a short time. This device is covered by insurance in many cases but the use of it should be discussed with the child's physician first.

When lifestyle modifications fall short in bringing relief to the child, doctors will turn to medications that have been approved for children. Antacids can be used according to the doses prescribed for children by the physician. Pepcid (famotidine) and Zantac (ranitidine hydrochloride) are two H_2 RAs that have been approved for use in the pediatric population. Limited information on Tagamet (cimetidine) has been gathered in studies so it isn't recommended for children under the age of sixteen as of yet, according to the manufacturer's prescribing information; some doctors prescribe this, however. Currently, the safety and effectiveness of Axid (nizatidine) has not been established in the pediatric population. Some PPI medications, such as Prilosec and Prevacid, have been approved for use in the pediatric population; for children not yet trained to swallow pills, the capsules are generally opened and placed in applesauce or yogurt and consumed. Reglan (metoclopomide), the prokinetic agent, can be used but its side effects can make it intolerable for some children; domperidone, not currently available in the United States but available in Canada and Europe, has been shown to be beneficial and safe for children in appropriate doses.

In current medical circles, surgery is not generally seen as the best treatment for many children with GERD but perhaps may be the only viable option for a small percentage of them. Because many children outgrow the condition before toddlerhood and many more respond favorably to medical therapy, the feeling among physicians is to take a wait-and-see approach while attempting medical therapy. Additionally, those who would seem to gain the most from such techniques—children with respiratory symptoms or those with neurological dysfunction—appear in a few studies to suffer from more complications of the surgery, including having the wrap come undone and requiring further surgery.

That said, a small portion of pediatric patients do undergo surgical procedures, the laproscopic Nissen fundoplication being by far the most common. These small surgical candidates—some of whom have Barrett's esophagus, strictures, were born prematurely, have respiratory conditions or neurological disease—face the same side effects and recovery from the surgery as their adult counterparts.

Reflux in senior adulthood

THERE ARE PLENTY of signs and symptoms of aging that humans experience. Hair grays, wrinkles form, joints creak, bones thin, muscles weaken, among other things. While these changes may not be welcome in some, the common health reminders of age may be slightly more perplexing, particularly the rise in age-related diseases such as heart disease or diabetes.

Digestively, the body may also show signs of age as well. Diverticulum, small sacs that form predominantly in the wall of the colon, generally make their debut after the age of fifty. Colon cancer rates rise after the age of fifty, though the disease may make its appearance earlier in some individuals. Constipation often becomes an issue in older adults for a variety of reasons, including the effect of certain medications taken for other situations and the avoidance of fibrous foods due to dental problems.

Upper gastrointestinal problems may surface as well; in particular, the elderly population, those over the age of sixty-five, reports a greater incidence rate of GERD than their younger counterparts. The reasons for the rise in reflux are many and varied.

For one, weakened muscles and ligaments throughout the body occur as humans age. In the upper gastrointestinal tract, this can translate into a case of hiatal hernia, due to weakened ligaments that attach the esophagus to the diaphragm. This slackening can allow the stomach to herniate into the thoracic cavity. A few studies have shown that the presence of this complication increases with age, being most prevalent in those over the age of fifty-five. Further, muscles that make up the LES can lose tone, causing there to be less pressure to keep that juncture closed during and after digestion. To complicate matters, the breakdown of food and delivery of it to the stomach may be compromised by a number of issues as well. Many elderly individuals experience dental issues that affect the way in which food is chewed and others may experience a neurological disease such as Parkinson's or problem such as a stroke that makes swallowing more difficult.

Motility in general appears to be complicated by age, by some medications that are used for age-related conditions, or by the conditions themselves. Some research has indicated that some people experience a slowing of gastric motility as they age; a lesser number may experience it if they become bedridden due to illness or accident. For example, diabetes mellitus and Parkinson's disease are more prevalent in the elderly population and both are related to impaired gastric motility.

Many individuals in this age bracket also tend to take more medications than their younger counterparts to combat a variety of conditions; some of these medications can result in "dry mouth," the cottony feeling resulting from decreased production of saliva. Saliva not only contains enzymes to break down certain carbohydrates, but it also aids in washing acid from the esophagus to the stomach. Medications taken for age-related conditions—calcium channel blockers, alpha and beta antagonists for heart conditions, and a number of other medications—can reduce the tone of the LES, allowing for a greater chance of reflux. Also, taking more medications means there exists a greater potential for a pill getting stuck in the throat and potentially wearing away the mucosa on which it rests, a painful condition known as pill esophagitis.

To treat GERD in older adults, doctors first may look toward the most obvious and easiest changes that can be made to lessen symptoms. So trying certain lifestyle modifications such as drinking a full glass of water with medication, eating smaller evening meals, and raising the head of the bed will likely be attempted first. If certain LES-weakening medications are taken, physicians also may opt for similarly effective medications that don't carry that side effect.

An eye is also kept on economical solutions, as older adults may have restricted income and the cost of medication may be one of the most important factors doctors consider in prescribing. Because many seniors are on a fixed income, it may be more cost-effective for them to take the more moderately priced H_2 RAs rather than pricier PPIs. This doesn't mean that senior citizens don't take PPIs; rather, those who do likely have adequate savings or additional insurance that covers the costs of these medications.

Another factor that doctors take into consideration when prescribing medication to the elderly population is that this population may be more sensitive to its effects. As one example, there is a higher incidence rate of decreased renal function in the elderly population. Since certain medications, such as the H_2 RAs, are excreted through the kidneys, this can leave an unwelcome burden on this organ. These individuals may have to lower their doses of the medications in order to tolerate them. Other seniors may metabolize medications more slowly or be more sensitive to the side effects, leaving many doctors to alter the prescribed amount to achieve the desired effect without the side effects.

To complicate matters further, senior adults tend to have some of the worst complications of reflux, such as stricture formation, Barrett's esophagus, and esophagitis, usually due to long-standing reflux that went untreated in the past. Add to this the fact that pain sensitivity to the symptoms of heartburn may be decreased in the senior patient and you have a potential recipe for disaster. Because of these factors, doctors treating an elderly patient may suggest a more conservative approach to surveillance of the esophagus than they would in a younger patient, opting for more frequent endoscopic procedures to monitor any complications more carefully. While no one enjoys such procedures, it is usually best to follow the orders to catch any changes when they are still manageable.

Surgical treatment may not occur as often in this population as in the younger cohort. Just about any surgery for anyone in this age group automatically incurs greater risks than that done on younger adults. Healing times are longer in senior citizens than in their younger counterparts, and young adults rarely have complicating factors such as neurological conditions, heart disease, or diabetes to add to the risk and healing times. With regard to GERD surgery, sugrical procedures are usually done in those who do not want to take PPIs for extended periods of time, usually not a reasonable reason for surgery in the elderly. Instead, every effort is expended in keeping acid reflux to a minimum with medications and in monitoring complications on a regular basis to catch any changes at the earliest possible time.

PART 2

THE COOKBOOK

INTRODUCTION

THINK AN ACID reflux diet is opposed to interesting and delicious eating? Not so. As with any diet that involves food restrictions, creativity and ingredient substitutions can turn bland and boring into easy to prepare, appetizing, and downright delicious.

As a food writer and teacher, I long ago learned that while people like to look at and to learn about elaborate foods, those dishes they actually prepare on a regular basis are simple, homey, and comforting. To most, the best recipes are those you can eat often. These are not overly fussy dishes with a laundry list of unusual or hard-to-find ingredients. These are dishes you can actually make and enjoy often, full of fresh vegetables and fruits and staple supermarket components. For variety, many include multicultural flavors and seasonings.

The recipes included in this collection are those many Americans would like to eat if they could eat anything they wanted—if they didn't suffer afterward. In short, if you didn't know they were created to abate GERD, you would think they were "regular" recipes.

What's different? Popular trigger foods are eliminated, very limited, or optional, depending on your individual tolerance for these foods. If they're listed at all, they will carry the warning "as tolerated." Because it would be impossible to tailor a cookbook to each individual's reflux triggers, we have attempted to reduce the overall quantities of these ingredients throughout the cookbook. Where a recipe in a normal cookbook would call for, say, a half of a cup of balsamic vinegar, we may have three tablespoons; even then, the "as tolerated" allows you to reduce this amount to taste.

One also has to take into account just how much of the ingredient is contained in the total recipe. You may see, for example, three tablespoons of vinegar, but it is combined with three cups or a couple of pounds of other ingredients; in other words, the potentially offending ingredient has been reduced significantly so as to add flavor but reduce the chance of reflux.

You will also not find a recipe that is deep fried or particularly fatty. This is for a couple of reasons. Fatty foods are, of course, reflux triggers, but they are also very caloric, which helps pack on the pounds. If you're overweight, these low-fat recipes will help you stay on course.

I repeat what Jill wrote in chapter 3: portion size is important, especially for people with GERD. The portions here are very satisfying, but they're based on three meals a day, not the smaller quantities you may eat more often because of your reflux. This is because you will most likely share these recipes with individuals who don't share your particular health concerns regarding reflux triggers, such as portion size. If a recipe serves six, you could very well serve eight. Use your judgment when figuring how much you should eat.

—Annabel Cohen

Solving GERD food issues

SIMPLY THINKING ABOUT some spices can bring on fear in many people. GERD sufferers often take drastic approaches to diet, because they often put the blame on entire categories of food. Add this to the fact that GERD can be exacerbated by factors discussed in chapter 3, and the food flavor outlook can be bleak.

While it's true that some foods are known triggers—stimulating production of acid or relaxing the LES—not every trigger affects every person. This is good news. While some may tolerate garlic, others may find even small amounts of it has troubling effects. Some can eat it for lunch, but not for dinner. Some people can tolerate cooked trigger foods, but not raw. Onions are a good example. Some people can eat them raw but not cooked, others can tolerate shallots but not scallions (both varieties of onions), while others must avoid them entirely. With other common triggers such as citrus or tomatoes, some find they can drink fresh-squeezed orange juice or eat raw tomatoes, but not the processed or cooked variety. Some people can't touch a chili pepper without feeling a pain in their gullet, but bell peppers, having far less intensity, won't cause a problem at all. The lesson here is that every case is different.

There's a simple way to figure out what and how much hurts you: Do what mothers do with babies to test for food allergies. Introduce trigger foods into your diet one at a time and note symptoms. Prepare something simple, like plain mashed potatoes. Add a small amount of raw or cooked garlic to the potatoes. Using a notebook, start a food diary and write down exactly how much garlic you added. Eat these potatoes for lunch. Wait. You'll know soon enough if garlic triggers your GERD.

Repeat this exercise, writing everything down, with all the trigger foods. Do it twice a day, every day until you have figured out those foods you can tolerate and those you can't and at which point of the day those foods can be consumed safely. After all, some can eat early and feel fine, since they're sitting or standing most of the day and not bending too often or lying down. Unfortunately, others may not be able to tolerate any trigger foods, no matter what position they are in or what time of the day it is. Write in your diary how you feel after consuming the food and you'll know for sure. Only then can you make educated decisions about what works—and doesn't work—for you. On a separate note, if you're overweight, losing weight may be enough to allow you eat most anything (see chapter 3 regarding weight loss and GERD).

The following is a list of common trigger foods and spices you'll want to test and ultimately avoid if they bother you. Your list may be longer or shorter. Find out for yourself.

Food and spices

Allspice
Black pepper
Chili peppers
Chili powder
Chocolate
Cinnamon
Citrus (limes, lemons, oranges, grapefruit, etc.)
Cucumbers
Curry
Garlic (raw, cooked, powder, salt)
Horseradish (raw, prepared)
Mustard
Nutmeg
Onions (cooked, raw)
Peppermint
Radishes
Sugar
Tomatoes
Vinegar
And high-fat, fried, or deep-fried foods

Beverages

Alcohol
Caffeinated drinks
Carbonated drinks
Coffee
Grapefruit juice (fresh squeezed may be better)
Orange juice (fresh squeezed may be better)
Tea, nonherbal
Tomato juice

Change your ways!

YOU ARE ON a learning path now, rediscovering what works for you. What you may figure out now is that you will have to prepare most of the food you consume. For some, that is not such a huge leap, but for others who don't know a frying pan from a saucepan, this may be a daunting task. Trust me. You can do it.

Modifying your cooking style is not difficult, even if you're not a talented cook. Most recipes—even baked goods—can be easily tailored to your needs. A good place to start in your cooking modification is in fat reduction. Often, recipes contain a larger amount of fat than necessary.

Initially, **buy yourself a good set of nonstick cookware.** Fat makes food not stick to the bottom and sides of pots and pans. Nonstick cooking surfaces are just that, so you don't need the fat to keep food from scorching. Most recipes are not compromised by cutting fat. Better yet, cut the fat completely, if possible. Don't worry about not having enough fat in your diet. Many foods and vegetables have enough natural fat in them to fulfill the need for fats in your diet.

The same is true for sugar. Many recipes simply contain too much sugar. **Start by cutting the sugar by a third the first time you make a recipe and then half the next time.** You'll acquire the taste for foods that are less sweet. It is possible. Although sugar substitutes often don't work in baked goods, there are new non-sugar products that are being introduced each year that promise success in baking. Keep your eyes open and be brave enough to try them. It is only through these challenges that we grow—and your recipe selection will grow, too.

Next, **learn to use nonstick cooking sprays to spray in cookware and even on your barbecue grill.** Use them to spray over foods instead of brushing oil or butter on top. Nonstick sprays come in many flavors so you'll have a nice selection from which to choose.

Lastly, **try substituting lower fat and nonfat ingredients for their fat-laden counterparts.** Mayonnaise, sour cream, half-and-half, cream cheese, cottage cheese, cheese in general, and salad dressings, among others, all have low-fat and nonfat counterparts.

The following lists foods to substitute. It's by no means complete, but will be of benefit when converting your favorite recipes. There are no substitutes for some foods. Zucchini will never replace tomatoes in marinara or other tomato-based pasta sauces, but they add to texture and flavor in other cooked foods in which tomatoes are usually added. And garlic's flavor is distinct, so there is no replacing that. Try drastically reducing the amount in recipes, substituting other palatable spices, or eliminating it altogether. It is a flavoring, so in nearly every case it doesn't affect food texture or consistency.

For these ingredients . . .	*Substitute these ingredients . . .*
Dairy—whole fat	Reduced-fat or nonfat dairy
Raw or cooked tomatoes	Raw or steamed zucchini
Fat in baking	Pureed fruit (like unsweetened applesauce)
Eggs	Two egg whites for each whole egg
Black pepper	Fresh or dried herbs
Cocoa powder	Carob powder (available at health food stores)
Chocolate chips	Butterscotch or peanut butter chips
Vinegar	Light soy sauce
Wine	Fat-free chicken stock or broth
Cinnamon	Allspice or nutmeg
Allspice	Cinnamon or nutmeg
Nutmeg	Cinnamon or allspice
Garlic, horseradish	Fresh or dried herbs

GREAT STARTERS

THE DIFFERENCE BETWEEN appetizers and hors d'oeuvres is only one of language. "Hors d'oeuvres" literally means "before the main work." But on occasion, hors d'oeuvres are the main work, or close to it.

Appetizers must be, well, appetizing. They should welcome and entice guests with flavors and aromas that pique the appetite if a full meal follows or satisfy hunger pangs if they're the sole offering. They allow for flavor experimentation and variety that may be absent from the main course. Mixing tastes and ethnic foods can prove quite successful. That's because small bites aren't meant to fill, just tease the palate.

The problem with appetizers and hors d'oeuvres is that often they're quite spicy—with hot peppers, garlic, and onions—and full of fat—deep fried or bathed in oil or butter. For anyone with GERD, appetizers are often forbidden. One small garlic-filled appetizer can mean hours of reflux. The following appetite teasers retain the savory flavors of your favorite starters while tempering or eliminating offensive GERD triggers.

It's good to know, too, that many of these appetizers can be made ahead, frozen, and reheated when you need them. Other appetizers can be made or prepped a day or two ahead and assembled just before serving. The less you have to do at the last moment, the better.

OLIVE AND ROASTED PEPPER CROSTINI

An APPETIZER YOU can make in a hurry, these crostini are delicious as appetizers, to serve with soup or salad or anytime you need a quick snack. They exclude reflux triggers like tomatoes and garlic, yet still retain the flavors that make these such a popular appetizer choice. For variety, add ingredients, change ingredients, and develop your own repertoire of crostini.

1 French or whole grain baguette
½ cup extra virgin olive oil
1 cup Kalamata olives, pitted and chopped
2 roasted red or yellow bell peppers
1 cup fresh grated or shredded Asiago cheese
Fresh chopped parsley, garnish
Whole basil leaves, garnish

1. Preheat oven to 350° F. Spray a baking sheet with nonstick cooking spray. Set aside.
2. Brush bread rounds with olive oil. Sprinkle remaining ingredients except basil over the rounds and place on the prepared baking sheet.
3. Bake for 10 minutes until the edges of the breads are crunchy and the topping is hot. Garnish with fresh basil leaves.

MAKES 30–40 CROSTINI ROUNDS.

NUTRIENT ANALYSIS PER SERVING:

Calories (kcal) 82 ■ Protein (g) 2.3 ■ Carbohydrates (g) 7.5 ■ Fat (g) 4.7 ■ Saturated Fat (g) 1 ■ Sodium (mg) 152 ■ Cholesterol (mg) 2.8 ■ % Calories from Protein 11 ■ % Calories from Carbohydrates 37 ■ % Calories from Fat 52 ■ Total Dietary Fiber (g) 0.7

Smoked Salmon on Black Bread Rounds with Mustard Dill Sauce

An almost instant appetizer, since this is more an assembly job than a cooking job. Smoked salmon is naturally salty, so the mayonnaise sauce tones down the flavor. Both mayonnaise and mustard usually contain vinegar, a known trigger. The amounts, however, are small, so you may not react to them. If in doubt, serve the appetizer without the sauce.

> *¼ cup nonfat mayonnaise*
> *1 tablespoon Dijon-style mustard*
> *2 tablespoons minced fresh dill*
> *1 package (12 ounces) pumpernickel party breads*
> *1 pound smoked salmon or lox, presliced, finely chopped*
> *Small sprigs of fresh dill for garnish*

1. Make the sauce: In a small bowl, stir together the mayonnaise, mustard, and dill until combined. Set aside.
2. Cut the party bread squares into star, heart, or circle shapes with a cookie cutter, or leave them whole, uncut. Place the breads on a serving tray.
3. Evenly divide and spread the mayonnaise mixture among the bread slices.
4. Place a small amount of the chopped salmon in the center of each bread slice. Garnish each appetizer with a small dill sprig.

Makes 3 dozen.

Nutrient Analysis Per Serving:

Calories (kcal) 40 ■ Protein (g) 3 ■ Carbohydrates (g) 4.7 ■ Fat (g) 1 ■ Saturated Fat (g) 0 ■ Sodium (mg) 178 ■ Cholesterol (mg) 3 ■ % Calories from Protein 32 ■ % Calories from Carbohydrates 48 ■ % Calories from Fat 20 ■ Total Dietary Fiber (g) .6

BAKED SPRING ROLLS

Deep fried spring rolls often have more fried crust than filling. Not these, made with super-thin rice paper. The paper merely holds the filling together, a nice change from the doughy Chinese-restaurant type. And they're considerably less caloric because they're baked, not fried.

> 3 ounces thin rice noodles (vermicelli, available in Asian markets)
> ½ teaspoon sesame oil
> 1 tablespoon white sesame seeds
> ½ cup grated or shredded carrots
> ½ cup fresh or canned water chestnuts, drained and sliced thin
> ½ cup thinly sliced pea pods
> 1 cup finely shredded green cabbage
> 2 teaspoons minced fresh gingerroot
> 1 tablespoon light soy sauce
> 1 tablespoon olive oil
> Warm water
> 8–12 large (8- or 9-inch diameter) rice paper rounds (available in
>   Asian markets)

1. Preheat oven to 400° F. Spray a cookie or baking sheet with nonstick cooking spray. Set aside.
2. Bring a medium pot of water to a boil over high heat. Add the rice noodles and boil for about 2 minutes or according to package directions. Drain well and transfer the noodles to a large bowl.
3. Add sesame oil, sesame seeds, carrots, water chestnuts, pea pods, cabbage, gingerroot, and soy sauce. Toss well to combine. Set aside.
4. Pour olive oil in a small bowl. Set aside.
5. Fill another shallow bowl with very warm water. Float a sheet of the rice paper in the water and submerge it gently with your fingers for about 20–30 seconds, until the paper is just softened. Remove from water and place on a clean surface. Gently brush the rice paper with a little olive oil.
6. Spoon ¼-cup of the filling onto rice paper edge closest to you. Fold the filling-lined edge of the rice paper over once. Fold the sides of the rice paper over the filling and roll up the rice paper like a thick cigar.

7. Place the roll, seam side down, on the prepared baking sheet. Spray the top of the roll with the nonstick cooking spray. Repeat with remaining filling and wrappers.

8. Bake the spring rolls, uncovered, for about 20 minutes, turning once or twice, until golden. Serve hot.

MAKES 8–12 SERVINGS.

───── **NUTRIENT ANALYSIS PER SERVING:** ─────

Calories (kcal) 108 ■ Protein (g) 2 ■ Carbohydrates (g) 19.5 ■ Fat (g) 2 ■ Saturated Fat (g) 0 ■ Sodium (mg) 151 ■ Cholesterol (mg) 1.4 ■ % Calories from Protein 8 ■ % Calories from Carbohydrates 73 ■ % Calories from Fat 19 ■ Total Dietary Fiber (g) 1.4

SUMMER ROLLS

Most of the ingredients here are available these days at the supermarket. If there are some you can't find, look to an Asian specialty market for them. Some people call these spring rolls and others call them fresh rolls; I've heard them called all three. No matter what you call them, they're fresh, delicious, and practically fat- and calorie-free. Plus there are really no GERD triggers in this recipe. Perfect for a light lunch or appetizer.

ROLLS:

3 ounces thin rice noodles (vermicelli)
8–12 large (8- or 9-inch diameter) rice paper rounds (available in
    Asian markets)
Warm water
8–10 large Boston or Bibb lettuce leaves
1 cup shredded carrots
Half large cucumber, seeded and cut into matchsticks
1½ cups fresh mung bean sprouts
¼ cup fresh mint leaves
½ cup fresh cilantro leaves
8 large boiled shrimp, cut in half lengthwise

1. Spread out all the ingredients in front of you. This is an assembly project.
2. Bring a pot of water to a boil over high heat. Add the noodles and cook for 2 minutes. Drain and rinse with cold water. Drain again very well. Set aside.
3. Stack several paper towels next to your workspace. Fill a shallow dish large enough to accommodate the rice paper rounds with warm water. Place one round in the water and let it soak until it is softened, 30–45 seconds.
4. Carefully remove the round with your fingers, being careful not to tear the round. Place the round on the paper towel to drain.
5. Move the rice paper round to your work surface and place a leaf of lettuce over the round. Add some noodles, carrots, cucumber, bean sprouts, and mint leaves to the lettuce and begin rolling the round. Roll the round halfway and add a few leaves of cilantro and two shrimp halves, cut sides up, on the round, and finish rolling tightly.
6. Cut the roll in half. Place the roll on a serving dish and cover with a damp cloth. Repeat with remaining ingredients and rice paper rounds. Makes 8 to 10 rolls

(depending on how full you make each one). Serve with hoisin peanut sauce, recipe below.

HOISIN PEANUT SAUCE:

½ cup hoisin sauce (available in Asian markets or well-stocked super-markets)

2 tablespoons creamy peanut butter

¼ cup water

2 tablespoons roasted peanuts, chopped

1. Combine all ingredients except peanuts in a small saucepan over medium-high heat.
2. Bring to a boil. Remove from heat and let cool.
3. To serve, pour into a small bowl and garnish with the chopped peanuts.

MAKES ABOUT 1 CUP OF SAUCE.

─────── NUTRIENT ANALYSIS PER SERVING: ───────

Calories (kcal) 181 ■ Protein (g) 6 ■ Carbohydrates (g) 30 ■ Fat (g) 4 ■ Saturated Fat (g) .7 ■ Sodium (mg) 406 ■ Cholesterol (mg) 13 ■ % Calories from Protein 13 ■ % Calories from Carbohydrates 67 ■ % Calories from Fat 21 ■ Total Dietary Fiber (g) 2.3

SMOKED BLUEFISH PATÉ

THE BLUEFISH IS wonderful on its own, and when mixed with cream cheese and a bit of horseradish, makes a wonderful spread. Most fish spreads contain butter, which is full of fat and calories. This lightened version has no added fat (the fish has natural fat). Serve the paté in a small bowl with carrot sticks, black bread, or crackers for dipping or spreading. Or use a small one- or two-ounce portion scoop to put a little on each guest's bread plate to serve instead of butter.

> 8 ounces smoked bluefish, skin and bones removed
> 4 ounces nonfat cream cheese
> 2 tablespoons fat-free evaporated milk
> 1 teaspoon white horseradish (as tolerated)

1. Combine all ingredients in the bowl of a food processor. Process until smooth.
2. Transfer the mixture to a small serving bowl. Serve with carrot sticks or gourmet crackers.

MAKES I CUP OF PATÉ.

NUTRIENT ANALYSIS PER SERVING:

Calories (kcal) 66 ■ Protein (g) 10 ■ Carbohydrates (g) 2.5 ■ Fat (g) 1.5 ■ Saturated Fat (g) 0 ■ Sodium (mg) 94 ■ Cholesterol (mg) 23 ■ % Calories from Protein 58 ■ % Calories from Carbohydrates 16 ■ % Calories from Fat 21 ■ Total Dietary Fiber (g) 0

Baba Ganouche

A MIDDLE EASTERN favorite that's made less caloric with eggplant instead of the chickpea version called hummus. Tahini (sesame seed paste) is quite caloric, but in small amounts acceptable for GERD sufferers. While garlic is typically included in large amounts, the quantity has been reduced. If you have reactions to even small amounts of garlic, leave it out. Lemon juice or vinegar, another traditional ingredient, and reflux trigger, has been eliminated entirely.

1 medium eggplant, unpeeled
¼ cup tahini
1 teaspoon chopped fresh garlic (as tolerated)
½ teaspoon ground cumin
Salt to taste
2 tablespoons extra virgin olive oil
12 Kalamata olives, garnish

1. Preheat oven to 400° F.
2. Use the tines of a fork to prick eggplant in at least 12 places. Place the eggplant in a shallow baking dish or on a baking sheet and roast it, uncovered, for about 1 hour, turning every 10 minutes or so, until very tender and soft to the touch.
3. Remove the eggplant from the oven and allow it to cool enough to touch.
4. Cut the eggplant in half lengthwise, and use a spoon to scoop out and scrape the eggplant pulp from its skin.
5. Discard skin and transfer the pulp to the bowl of a food processor. Add remaining ingredients, except olive oil and olives, and pulse until just combined with a slightly chunky texture (do not puree).
6. Spoon the mixture into a shallow bowl and drizzle with olive oil. Arrange the olives around the edge of the bowl. Serve the spread with pita wedges or raw vegetables.

MAKES 2 CUPS OF BABA GANOUCHE, ABOUT 8 SERVINGS.

NUTRIENT ANALYSIS PER SERVING:

Calories (kcal) 110 ▪ Protein (g) 3 ▪ Carbohydrates (g) 5 ▪ Fat (g) 9 ▪ Saturated Fat (g) 0.5 ▪ Sodium (mg) 95 ▪ Cholesterol (mg) 0 ▪ % Calories from Protein 10 ▪ % Calories from Carbohydrates 19 ▪ % Calories from Fat 74 ▪ Total Dietary Fiber (g) 2

TAPENADE

A FRENCH STARTER made with olives as its main ingredient. A little goes a long way with tapenade because the flavor is quite strong. Most varieties of olives are not GERD triggers. Although the recipe calls for mayonnaise, which often includes vinegar, the amount of vinegar is just a small percentage of the mayonnaise. Serve tapenade as a spread for small breads or as a dip for raw vegetables.

> *4 anchovy fillets (as tolerated)*
> *2 cups Kalamata or Italian black olives or other oil-cured olives, pitted*
> *1 tablespoon Worcestershire sauce*
> *¼ cup fresh parsley*
> *½ cup nonfat mayonnaise*
> *¼ teaspoon minced garlic (as tolerated)*

1. In a food processor fitted with a metal blade, combine the anchovies, olives, Worcestershire sauce, and parsley. Pulse until chopped and combined, but not a paste.
2. Transfer the mixture to a bowl and fold in the mayonnaise.
3. Serve as a spread for French bread rounds or gourmet crackers. Alternately, you may serve a small amount of tapenade spooned on the cut ends of Belgian endive leaves as a passed appetizer.

MAKES 2 CUPS.

NUTRIENT ANALYSIS PER SERVING:

Calories (kcal) 55 ▪ Protein (g) 1 ▪ Carbohydrates (g) 4.7 ▪ Fat (g) 3.8 ▪ Saturated Fat (g) .5 ▪ Sodium (mg) 508 ▪ Cholesterol (mg) 1.7 ▪ % Calories from Protein 7 ▪ % Calories from Carbohydrates 34 ▪ % Calories from Fat 62 ▪ Total Dietary Fiber (g) 1

ZUCCHINI AND SUN-DRIED TOMATO CROSTINI

HERE IS ANOTHER version of this famous Italian appetizer that's always made with small toast rounds. Infinitely variable to your own taste, crostini is among the simplest of appetizers to prepare. This recipe includes sun-dried tomatoes, though, which, even in a small amount, may trigger GERD. If you're very sensitive to the tomatoes, leave them off the crostini or substitute another ingredient—such as chopped artichoke hearts—for the tomatoes.

> 3 cups ½-inch diced zucchini
> 1 French or whole grain baguette or whole grain bread or rolls, sliced
>   into thin (¼-inch) rounds
> 3 tablespoons olive oil
> ½ cup sun-dried tomatoes, drained and chopped
> ¼ cup fresh chopped basil
> ¼ cup fresh chopped parsley
> Kosher salt to taste
> ½ cup freshly grated Parmesan cheese, garnish

1. Preheat oven to 350° F. Spray a baking sheet with nonstick cooking spray. Set aside.
2. Heat oil in a large skillet over medium-high heat. Add zucchini and cook for 5 minutes, stirring occasionally, until the zucchini are very soft. Allow to cool for a few minutes.
3. Brush bread rounds with olive oil. Sprinkle zucchini and remaining ingredients over the rounds and place on the prepared baking sheet.
4. Bake for 10 minutes until the edges of the breads are crunchy and the topping is hot.

MAKES 30–40 CROSTINI ROUNDS.

NUTRIENT ANALYSIS PER SERVING:

Calories (kcal) 54 ▪ Protein (g) 1.7 ▪ Carbohydrates (g) 7.2 ▪ Fat (g) 2.0 ▪ Saturated Fat (g) 0.5 ▪ Sodium (mg) 108 ▪ Cholesterol (mg) .9 ▪ % Calories from Protein 13 ▪ % Calories from Carbohydrates 53 ▪ % Calories from Fat 34 ▪ Total Dietary Fiber (g) 0.6

Sesame Chicken Satays with Peanut Sauce

Asatay is a kebab by any other name. This version is sweet and savory with a distinct Asian flavor. If you're in a hurry, use plain Hoisin sauce as the dipping sauce. The recipe includes small amounts of red wine vinegar and garlic, big reflux triggers. Though the amount is small, you may wish to exclude the vinegar altogether. The peanut sauce contains calming gingerroot.

> *1 tablespoon sesame oil*
> *2 tablespoons olive oil*
> *1 tablespoon red wine vinegar (as tolerated)*
> *3 tablespoons light soy sauce*
> *2 tablespoons brown sugar*
> *¼ cup sesame seeds*
> *1 pound boneless, skinless chicken breasts, washed, patted dry, cut into*
>   *½-inch chunks*

Peanut sauce:

> *3 tablespoons olive oil*
> *¼ teaspoon minced garlic (as tolerated)*
> *2 tablespoons fresh, chopped gingerroot*
> *½ cup creamy peanut butter*
> *1 tablespoon red wine vinegar (as tolerated)*
> *2 tablespoons light soy sauce*
> *1 tablespoon sugar*
> *¼ cup warm water or more as needed*

1. In a medium bowl, whisk together the sesame and olive oils, vinegar, soy sauce, brown sugar, and sesame seeds.
2. Add the chicken chunks and marinate, chilled, for at least 30 minutes or up to 2 hours.
3. Meanwhile, to prepare the peanut sauce, place all of the sauce ingredients except water in the bowl of a food processor and process until smooth. Add warm water as necessary to thin the sauce if it is too thick to be used as a dipping sauce. Set aside.
4. Preheat the oven to 350° F.

5. Thread 2–3 chunks of chicken onto a round toothpick and place on a baking sheet. Repeat with remaining chicken. Discard remaining marinade.

6. Bake for 8–10 minutes until just cooked through. Serve warm or at room temperature with peanut sauce on the side.

MAKES 30 APPETIZERS.

NUTRIENT ANALYSIS PER SERVING:

Calories (kcal) 82 ■ Protein (g) 5 ■ Carbohydrates (g) 3 ■ Fat (g) 5.8 ■ Saturated Fat (g) 1 ■ Sodium (mg) 119 ■ Cholesterol (mg) 9 ■ % Calories from Protein 24 ■ % Calories from Carbohydrates 14 ■ % Calories from Fat 64 ■ Total Dietary Fiber (g) .4

SPINACH-AND FETA-STUFFED PHYLLO SHELLS

A QUICK VERSION of spinach pie or triangles, this recipe deletes reflux triggers onions and garlic. It also cuts way down on the fat that's usually used with phyllo dough and in the filling ingredients. Phyllo, or filo dough as it is sometimes spelled, can be difficult to work with, since it dries out very quickly. These premade tiny pastry shells are available in the frozen food department of well-stocked supermarkets. They are a wonderful shortcut ingredient, served filled with just about anything.

1 package (10 ounces) frozen chopped spinach, thawed, well drained
   and squeezed to remove excess water
¼ cup crumbled feta cheese
¼ cup fat-free cottage cheese
¼ cup grated Parmesan cheese
4 egg whites
2 tablespoons fresh chopped dill or 1 tablespoon dried dill
2 packages frozen, premade, mini phyllo shells (about 30 shells)

1. Preheat the oven to 325° F. Spray a baking sheet with nonstick cooking spray.
2. In a medium bowl, combine the spinach, feta, cottage and Parmesan cheeses, egg whites, and dill. Divide the mixture evenly among the frozen phyllo cups and place the cups on the prepared baking sheet.
3. Bake for 15–20 minutes until the phyllo is golden and the filling is hot.

MAKES 30 APPETIZERS.

NUTRIENT ANALYSIS PER SERVING:

Calories (kcal) 35 ■ Protein (g) 2 ■ Carbohydrates (g) 3 ■ Fat (g) 1.5 ■ Saturated Fat (g) .3 ■ Sodium (mg) 57 ■ Cholesterol (mg) 1.6 ■ % Calories from Protein 22 ■ % Calories from Carbohydrates 35 ■ % Calories from Fat 39 ■ Total Dietary Fiber (g) 0

ROAST BEEF PINWHEELS

PRETTY TO LOOK at and simple to make, this is another of those dishes that's merely an assembly project. For variety, use turkey instead of beef and add a few dried cranberries to the filling. While the mayonnaise contains vinegar, a GERD trigger, the amount is very small. Monterey Jack cheese is high in fat, though there are low-fat versions available. Since each roll contains only a couple of thin slices of cheese, the calories and fat are minimized.

1 8-ounce package fat-free cream cheese, softened
1 cup nonfat mayonnaise
½ cup horseradish, white or red
1 package large (at least 10 inches in diameter or more) lavash bread
*   (6–8 pieces) or favorite soft flatbread*
1 pound Monterey Jack cheese, very thinly sliced
1½ pounds good quality, lean, medium-rare roast beef, sliced thin
2 large red bell peppers, chopped
1–2 packages (about 4-ounces each) alfalfa sprouts

1. In a small bowl, stir together the cream cheese, mayonnaise, and horseradish until combined. Set aside.
2. Place one lavash on a clean, flat surface. Spread a thin layer of the cream cheese mixture over the bread, especially on the uppermost edge (this is the glue that holds the lavash together after it has been rolled).
3. Place about 2 slices of the cheese on the half of the lavash closest to you. Repeat with the roast beef. Sprinkle red peppers over the beef and place a large "line" of sprouts on top of the beef along the edge closest to you (this will end up in the center of the wrap).
4. Begin rolling from the edge closest to you, using your fingers to help keep the filling in place. The last turn of lavash should contain no filling.
5. Place the finished roll, seam side down, on a cutting board and cut the lavash, starting where the filling begins in the rolls, into approximately 1-inch slices. Repeat with the remaining lavash and filling. Discard the unfilled ends of lavash.

MAKES 40 OR MORE APPETIZERS.

NUTRIENT ANALYSIS PER SERVING:

Calories (kcal) 119 ■ Protein (g) 9.3 ■ Carbohydrates (g) 7 ■ Fat (g) 5.8 ■ Saturated Fat (g) 3 ■
Sodium (mg) 168 ■ Cholesterol (mg) 24 ■ % Calories from Protein 31 ■ % Calories from
Carbohydrates 24 ■ % Calories from Fat 44 ■ Total Dietary Fiber (g) 1

Satisfying Soups

It's not easy for GERD sufferers to find prepared soups that don't trigger reflux attacks. Because soup manufacturers are making soup to satisfy a variety of tastes, they often contain large amounts of tomato, onion, garlic, and sodium, not to mention fat and calories. Especially when it comes to creamy soups. Homemade soup offers the only solution for many.

Perhaps the best feature of most soups is that they start with water—fat-free, no calories, and filling. Perfect for those trying to lose weight as part of a GERD control. And they are basic and versatile. They can start a meal or be a meal. As starters, they foretell an entire meal experience. Thick or chunky soup is like a warm embrace; it reaches way down to comfort. And hot soup is an experience that lingers long after the meal is over. It's what was meant when they coined the phrase "sticks to the ribs." Cold soup will keep your temperature down in the heat and is as refreshing as a tall drink of water.

Soup making is not without tribulations. The uncertainty many cooks experience can come from fear of making flavorless soup. Some fear that the soups they make just won't taste good and if soup isn't good, you've wasted ingredients and admitted defeat.

The second issue is more a problem of time. While on television, professional chefs seem to chop, sauté, and throw in the exact, perfect amount of oregano, the nonpro may take a whole lot longer to gather ingredients and chop them without losing fingers. And how many people in the world have chicken or vegetable stock at their fingertips?

Help is on the way. The recipes listed here are contemporary—the kinds of soups you'd eat in trendy restaurants. The surprise is that these recipes usually take less than twenty minutes or so to prepare—including the chopping and dicing. All that's left after is the cooking time. And, with the exception of the bread soup, the soups here feed a crowd, not the one or two portions you can usually eke out of prepared cans and packages.

ROASTED VEGETABLE SOUP

ROASTING VEGETABLES ADDS flavor to this soup without adding GERD-offensive spices. It's extremely low in fat and full of fiber, so it's filling and perfect as part of a weight-loss regime. This soup is like a garden in a bowl. It's so refreshing served cold on a hot summer's evening and perfect served hot if you're not a cold soup fan. Cilantro is comforting for reflux sufferers. If you can tolerate the garlic and a bit of heat, add the garlic and hot pepper sauce. If not, leave them out.

> 2 tablespoons olive oil
> 2 zucchini, cut into ½-inch pieces
> 1 cup fresh or frozen corn kernels (thawed if using frozen)
> 10 thin asparagus stalks cut into ½-inch pieces or ¼ pound green beans
> 1 teaspoon minced fresh garlic (as tolerated)
> ½ teaspoon dried oregano
> ½ teaspoon ground cumin
> Salt to taste
> 5 cups water, fat-free chicken, or vegetable broth
> 1 tablespoon hot pepper sauce, such as Tabasco (as tolerated)
> 1 can (15-ounce) chickpeas or white beans
> 1 cup frozen peas, thawed
> ½ cup chopped fresh cilantro, loosely packed

1. Preheat oven to 450° F. Brush the olive oil lightly over the bottom of a large roasting pan.
2. Add zucchini, corn, asparagus, garlic (if using), oregano, cumin, and salt; toss well. Roast the vegetables, uncovered, for about 15–25 minutes, turning occasionally.
3. Remove from oven and cool completely. Transfer the vegetables to a large saucepan and add the broth, hot sauce, chickpeas, peas, and cilantro. Bring to a boil over high heat, reduce heat, and simmer for 30 minutes. Remove from heat and cool.
4. Chill, covered, until ready to serve, up to 2 days ahead. Add more water or broth if the soup is too thick for your taste. If serving hot, heat through and adjust salt to taste. Serve in bowls or mugs.

MAKES 8 SERVINGS.

NUTRIENT ANALYSIS PER SERVING:

Calories (kcal) 120 ■ Protein (g) 5 ■ Carbohydrates (g) 16 ■ Fat (g) 5 ■ Saturated Fat (g) 0.5 ■ Sodium (mg) 244 ■ Cholesterol (mg) 0 ■ % Calories from Protein 15 ■ % Calories from Carbohydrates 54 ■ % Calories from Fat 36 ■ Total Dietary Fiber (g) 4

HEARTY FISH CHOWDER IN BREAD BOWLS

A ONE-DISH meal, this hearty soup is fun to eat, because after you finish the soup, you eat the bowl. There are onions in the recipe, though not as many as in "regular" recipes for this type of soup, which can call for up to two cups of chopped onions! Don't be concerned about tomato paste, one of the great GERD offenders in this recipe. The small amount used will help make the soup red, but is negligible when diluted by the liquid in the soup. If dairy products cause you discomfort, feel free to use nondairy creamer in this recipe.

¼ cup olive oil
½ cup chopped onions (as tolerated)
2 cups diced carrots
1 cup diced celery
2 tablespoons flour
2 teaspoons sweet or mild paprika
4 cups fat-free chicken, broth, fish broth, or water
1 cup fat-free half-and-half
4 cups small diced potatoes, peeled or unpeeled
1–2 pounds fish, such as cod, salmon, halibut, etc., cut into large
  chunks or a combination (use shellfish, too, if you wish)
1 cup fresh or frozen peas (if using frozen, thaw first)
¼ cup fresh chopped parsley or 2 tablespoons dried
1 tablespoon tomato paste (as tolerated)
Kosher salt to taste
4–8 bread bowls, depending on the size of the bowls, tops cut off,
  insides mostly scooped out. Save the bread tops as "lids" for the
  bread bowls.

1. Heat oil in a soup pot over medium-high heat. Add the onions, if using, carrots, and celery and cook, stirring occasionally until the vegetables are softened.
2. Add flour and paprika and stir well to coat the vegetables. Cook for a few minutes, stirring occasionally. (The flour on the vegetables will thicken the soup.)
3. Add the broth, half-and-half, and potatoes. Bring the mixture to a boil, reduce the heat, and simmer the chowder, covered, for 15 minutes or until the potatoes are tender, stirring occasionally.

4. Add the fish, peas, parsley, and tomato paste, if using. Cook for 10 minutes more, until the fish is cooked through.
5. Season to taste with salt. Serve hot, ladled into the hollowed bread "bowls."

MAKES 6–10 SERVINGS, DEPENDING ON THE SIZE OF THE BREAD BOWLS.

NUTRIENT ANALYSIS PER SERVING:

Calories (kcal) 465 ■ Protein (g) 26 ■ Carbohydrates (g) 66 ■ Fat (g) 10.6 ■ Saturated Fat (g) 1.5 ■ Sodium (mg) 846 ■ Cholesterol (mg) 35.6 ■ % Calories from Protein 23 ■ % Calories from Carbohydrates 57 ■ % Calories from Fat 21 ■ Total Dietary Fiber (g) 9.4

EIGHT-VEGETABLE MINESTRONE

Low in fat, this minestrone will fill you up—with fiber and healthy vegetables. For this truly hearty soup, you can be as creative as you want, mixing in meat and chicken to add variety to the vegetables. The trick to the creamy texture of this soup is to blend or puree a portion of the soup to make it thicker. Just before serving, sprinkle the soup with fresh grated cheese, such as Parmesan or Romano. Like other minestrone recipes, this one includes onions and tomato paste. The difference is that these ingredients are used sparingly, as flavorings only.

¼ cup olive oil
½ cup chopped onions (as tolerated)
1 cup carrots, diced or cut into rings
½ cup celery, diced or sliced
1 cup diced turnips
1 cup diced potatoes
1 14-ounce can great northern or cannellini beans, drained
1 tablespoon tomato paste (as tolerated)
1 large can (about 48 ounces) fat-free chicken broth
2 tablespoons dried parsley flakes
1 cup diced zucchini
1 cup frozen peas, thawed
½ cup dry small pasta, such as macaroni, ziti, or shells
Kosher salt to taste
Fresh grated Parmesan or Romano cheese, garnish

1. Heat oil in a large pot over medium-high heat. Add the onions, if using, and cook, stirring frequently until they are softened, about 5 minutes.
2. Add the carrots, celery, turnips, potatoes, beans, tomato paste, and chicken broth and bring to a boil. Reduce heat to a low boil and cook the soup, covered, for 1 hour.
3. Let the soup cool slightly before blending or pureeing about 2 cups of the vegetables and a little broth until smooth, in the pitcher of a blender or the bowl of a food processor.
4. Pour the puree back into the soup pot and add the parsley, zucchini, peas, pasta, and salt.
5. Bring the soup to a boil over medium-high heat, reduce heat, and cook uncovered for about 15 minutes until the soup is very hot and thickened.

6. Adjust salt to taste and serve very hot with fresh grated cheese and warm crusty bread. The soup may also be served in bread bowls if desired.

Makes 8–12 hearty servings.

Nutrient Analysis Per Serving:

Calories (kcal) 166 ■ Protein (g) 9 ■ Carbohydrates (g) 17 ■ Fat (g) 7.2 ■ Saturated Fat (g) 1 ■ Sodium (mg) 322 ■ Cholesterol (mg) 15.2 ■ % Calories from Protein 21 ■ % Calories from Carbohydrates 40 ■ % Calories from Fat 39 ■ Total Dietary Fiber (g) 3.8

ROASTED MUSHROOM SOUP

ROASTING MUSHROOMS GIVES them a rich, earthy flavor that's a definite plus in this soup. The soup is not creamy or thick; rather, it's a fresh broth that's light and satisfying with significantly fewer calories and less sodium than commercial soups. If dairy products don't agree with you, use nondairy creamer instead.

> *1 pound white or button mushrooms*
> *½ pound shiitake or crimini mushrooms, tough stems removed*
> *1 tablespoon olive oil*
> *4 cups low sodium, fat-free chicken stock or broth*
> *2 cups ½-inch diced russet or Idaho potatoes*
> *1 cup fat-free evaporated milk*
> *⅛ teaspoon ground nutmeg*
> *Salt to taste*
> *Fresh chopped parsley or chives (as tolerated), garnish*

1. Preheat oven to 400° F. Clean mushrooms by wiping them well with a clean, damp cloth.
2. Toss the mushrooms with the oil in a roasting pan. Roast the mushrooms, uncovered, for 20 minutes.
3. Meanwhile bring the broth to a boil in a large saucepan over medium-high heat. Add potatoes and bring to a boil again. Reduce heat to a simmer and cook the potatoes for 10–15 minutes, until tender. Remove from heat and cool slightly.
4. Remove mushrooms from the oven and cool slightly.
5. Combine the mushrooms, potatoes, and broth in the pitcher of a blender or bowl of a food processor. Blend or process until smooth (you may need to do this in batches).
6. Transfer the soup back to the pan and add the milk, nutmeg, and salt to taste. Add more water or broth if the soup is too thick.
7. Heat the soup until very hot and serve.

MAKES 6 SERVINGS.

NUTRIENT ANALYSIS PER SERVING:

Calories (kcal) 144 ■ Protein (g) 12 ■ Carbohydrates (g) 14.7 ■ Fat (g) 5.4 ■ Saturated Fat (g) .65 ■ Sodium (mg) 222 ■ Cholesterol (mg) 18.2 ■ % Calories from Protein 34 ■ % Calories from Carbohydrates 41 ■ % Calories from Fat 34 ■ Total Dietary Fiber (g) 1.3

Winter Squash Soup

W INTER SQUASH IS every bit as comforting as potatoes, especially in this creamy soup. And it's chock full of antioxidants and fiber. Wine gives the soup complexity. Even though wine is acidic, it's only used in a small amount relative to the rest of the soup. If dairy products don't agree with you, use nondairy creamer instead.

3 tablespoons olive oil
½ cup chopped onions (as tolerated)
3 pounds peeled, cubed winter squash, seeds removed (acorn or butter-
nut are good choices, or you may use frozen pureed squash as a
base—use 3 10-ounce packages, thawed)
4 cups water, or chicken or vegetable broth
1 cup white wine
½ teaspoon nutmeg
Kosher salt to taste
½ cup fat-free evaporated milk (as tolerated)

1. Heat olive oil in a large saucepan or small soup pot over medium-high heat. Add onions, if using, and cook, stirring, for about 5 minutes until the onions are softened.
2. Add the squash, water, wine, nutmeg, and salt and bring to a boil.
3. Reduce the heat, cover, and cook the soup for about an hour or until the squash is very tender. (This is very important—if the squash is not very soft, the soup will not puree smoothly.)
4. Let the soup cool slightly and ladle it into the bowl of a food processor or the pitcher of a blender (you may need to do this in batches). Blend or process the soup until very smooth. Place the pureed soup in a clean pot and repeat the process until all the soup is pureed.
5. Adjust the salt to taste and reheat the soup until hot. Add evaporated milk into the soup before serving.

MAKES 8 SERVINGS.

NUTRIENT ANALYSIS PER SERVING:

Calories (kcal) 140 ■ Protein (g) 3 ■ Carbohydrates (g) 22.2 ■ Fat (g) 5.3 ■ Saturated Fat (g) 0.7 ■ Sodium (mg) 94 ■ Cholesterol (mg) 0.4 ■ % Calories from Protein 8 ■ % Calories from Carbohydrates 63 ■ % Calories from Fat 34 ■ Total Dietary Fiber (g) 2.7

Turkey and Wild Rice Soup

THIS IS GREAT day-after-Thanksgiving soup, or for anytime you want a meal in a bowl. Very low in fat and high in fiber, the soup gets most of its flavor from the combination of vegetables rather than reflux-unfriendly garlic and spices. If you have leftover turkey, you can make the broth in this soup with the turkey carcass. Just add water to the bones and boil for two hours. Strain the broth and use it in place of chicken broth.

2 tablespoons olive oil
¼ cup chopped onions (as tolerated)
1½ cups chopped celery stalks
1½ cups diced carrots
1 large red bell pepper, chopped
9 cups low sodium, fat-free chicken stock or broth
1 cup water
1 cup wild rice
3 cups diced cooked turkey
1 package (10-ounce) frozen chopped spinach, thawed
1 bay leaf
2 tablespoons dried parsley flakes
Salt to taste

1. Heat oil in heavy large pot over medium heat. Add onions, if using, celery, carrots, and red bell pepper and sauté until vegetables are cooked through, about 8 minutes.
2. Add broth, water, rice, turkey, spinach, bay leaf, and parsley and bring soup to a boil.
3. Reduce heat to medium-low; simmer for 45 minutes until the rice is tender. Add more liquid if needed. Season the soup to taste with salt and serve hot.

MAKES 8 SERVINGS.

NUTRIENT ANALYSIS PER SERVING:

Calories (kcal) 265 ▪ Protein (g) 28.4 ▪ Carbohydrates (g) 21 ▪ Fat (g) 7 ▪ Saturated Fat (g) 1 ▪ Sodium (mg) 389 ▪ Cholesterol (mg) 65 ▪ % Calories from Protein 43 ▪ % Calories from Carbohydrates 32 ▪ % Calories from Fat 25 ▪ Total Dietary Fiber (g) 4

BLACK BEAN SOUP

THICK, DARK, AND filling, black beans are a wonderful protein, and since they take longer for the body to digest, they leave you feeling full far longer. Though they do cause gas in the colon, this should not affect the LES. Cilantro is GERD-friendly, so add as much as you like. As a variation, you may use white or northern beans instead of black for this recipe. Or prepare a half recipe of each and ladle them next to each other in a bowl for black and white bean soup. If you can't tolerate the dairy in the sour cream, use nondairy sour cream or leave it out altogether.

> 2 cups dried black beans, sorted, washed, and drained
> Water
> 8 cups low sodium, fat-free chicken stock, broth, or water
> 1 teaspoon dried thyme
> ½ teaspoon ground cumin
> 1 teaspoon minced garlic (as tolerated)
> 1 red bell pepper, chopped
> ½ cup shredded carrots
> 2 bay leaves
> Salt to taste
> ¼ cup chopped cilantro, optional
> Fat-free sour cream, garnish (as tolerated)

1. Place the beans in a large bowl and cover with water. Soak them for 5 hours or overnight. Drain, rinse, and drain the beans well.
2. Place the drained beans in a large pot and add the broth, thyme, cumin, garlic (if using), bell pepper, carrots, bay leaves, and salt. Bring the liquid to a boil, reduce heat to a simmer, cover, and cook for 1½ hours, until the beans are tender, adding more liquid if the soup is too thick.
3. Adjust seasonings to taste and serve hot with a bit of cilantro and a dollop of sour cream.

MAKES 4–6 SERVINGS.

NUTRIENT ANALYSIS PER SERVING:

Calories (kcal) 359 ■ Protein (g) 29 ■ Carbohydrates (g) 53 ■ Fat (g) 3.6 ■ Saturated Fat (g) .3 ■ Sodium (mg) 449 ■ Cholesterol (mg) 40 ■ % Calories from Protein 32 ■ % Calories from Carbohydrates 59 ■ % Calories from Fat 9 ■ Total Dietary Fiber (g) 12.4

CHICKEN NOODLE SOUP

THE ULTIMATE IN comfort, chicken noodle soup is claimed to be "penicillin" by at least four ethnic groups that I know of. Normally, chicken soup contains a large amount of onions, for both flavor and the golden color the onion skins add to the broth. We've left out the onion, but included all of the other ingredients necessary for good chicken soup. This soup calls for wide noodles, but cooked rice, barley, indeed any cooked grain, pasta, or dumpling is wonderful in this soup. For added fiber, try using whole-wheat pasta instead of regular noodles.

1 ¾ pound chicken, cut into pieces
3 quarts water
2 cups 2-inch carrot pieces
1 cup 2-inch parsnip pieces
1 cup 2-inch turnip pieces
1 cup chopped celery
1 cup diced celery
1 cup parsley sprigs
¼ cup fresh dill, uncut
Salt to taste
1 bay leaf
8 ounces dry extra-wide noodles
2 medium carrots, peeled and cut into ¼-inch rounds.

1. Combine chicken and water in a large pot; bring to a boil. Cook for 10 minutes and skim the foam or scum from the surface.
2. Add remaining ingredients, except noodles and carrot rounds, and bring to a boil again. Reduce heat to a low boil, cover, and cook the soup for 1½ hours, adding more water as needed.
3. Remove the soup from the heat and strain, removing the chicken and discarding the remaining ingredients.
4. Allow the chicken to cool and remove meat, discarding the skin and bones. Cut the chicken into ½-inch pieces and add the strained broth. Cool the soup and chill, covered overnight.

5. Remove the chilled, hardened fat from the soup and discard. Bring the soup to a boil over high heat, adding the noodles, carrot rounds, and salt to taste. Reduce heat, and simmer 10–15 minutes until the carrots are tender, adding more liquid if the soup is too condensed. Serve hot.

MAKES 8 SERVINGS.

NUTRIENT ANALYSIS PER SERVING:

Calories (kcal) 362 ■ Protein (g) 43.5 ■ Carbohydrates (g) 22 ■ Fat (g) 9.7 ■ Saturated Fat (g) 2 ■ Sodium (mg) 458 ■ Cholesterol (mg) 150 ■ % Calories from Protein 48 ■ % Calories from Carbohydrates 24 ■ % Calories from Fat 24 ■ Total Dietary Fiber (g) 1.2

MUSHROOM BARLEY SOUP

THIS DELI STAPLE is yet another soup that's thick and hearty. This recipe has been adapted to be much less of a reflux inciter, with onions and garlic greatly reduced. Though there's sherry in the recipe, it's minimal compared to the ten cups of other liquids in the recipe. It's also very low in fat and calories, for those watching their weight.

> 3 tablespoons olive oil
> 1/2 cup medium onions, chopped fine (as tolerated)
> 1/2 teaspoon minced garlic (as tolerated)
> 2 pounds white mushrooms, sliced thin
> 1 tablespoon soy sauce
> 1/2 cup medium-dry sherry
> 5 cups fat-free chicken broth
> 5 cups water
> 1 cup dry pearl barley
> 8 carrots, sliced diagonally into 1/4-inch-thick slices
> 1/2 teaspoon dried thyme
> 1/2 teaspoon dried rosemary
> 2 tablespoons dried parsley flakes
> Salt to taste

1. Heat oil in a large pot over medium-high heat. Add onions and garlic and cook for 3 minutes.
2. Add mushrooms and soy sauce and sauté over moderately high heat, stirring, until liquid the mushrooms release is almost evaporated.
3. Add sherry and cook, stirring occasionally, until evaporated.
4. Add broth, water, barley, carrots, and dried herbs to mushroom mixture and simmer, uncovered, 1 hour, adding more liquid if needed.
5. Season soup with salt to taste and serve hot.

MAKES 8 SERVINGS.

NUTRIENT ANALYSIS PER SERVING:

Calories (kcal) 234 ■ Protein (g) 11 ■ Carbohydrates (g) 30.6 ■ Fat (g) 8.4 ■ Saturated Fat (g) 1 ■ Sodium (mg) 332 ■ Cholesterol (mg) 15.6 ■ % Calories from Protein 19 ■ % Calories from Carbohydrates 52 ■ % Calories from Fat 33 ■ Total Dietary Fiber (g) 6.8

Bread Soup

This soup is inspired by "sopa seca"—the so-called dry soup of Portugal, named for the dry bread that's the chief ingredient. There's a small amount of tomato sauce in this recipe for color and flavor, but not so much as to cause GERD. There's also a handful of cilantro, included for its exotic taste and soothing ability. The poached egg on top has a runny yolk that's stirred into the soup at the table. If you feel the poached egg idea isn't for you, slice hardboiled eggs or egg whites, if you're watching cholesterol, into the soup. It's still delicious that way.

> *4 cups ½-inch bread cubes from rustic or grainy bread, slightly dried*
> *¼ cup, or more, extra virgin olive oil*
> *½ cup chopped cilantro*
> *5 cups water, or fat-free chicken or vegetable broth*
> *2 tablespoons tomato sauce (as tolerated)*
> *2 tablespoons dried parsley flakes*
> *Salt to taste*
> *4 large eggs*

1. Prepare the bread cubes: Preheat oven to 350° F. Toss the cubes with the olive oil and place in one layer on a baking sheet. Bake the cubes for 10–15 minutes until golden.
2. Meanwhile, combine cilantro, broth, tomato sauce, parsley, and salt in a large saucepan over medium-high heat. Bring to a boil and simmer for five minutes while you poach the eggs.
3. Heat an egg-poacher or pot filled with 2 inches of water over high heat and bring to a boil.
4. Reduce heat to simmering, break one egg in a bowl, and gently slide it into the water. Repeat with remaining eggs. Let the eggs poach for 3-4 minutes until the whites are set, occasionally spooning some water over the top of the egg.
5. Meanwhile, divide the bread cubes evenly among four soup bowls.
6. Pour the soup over the bread cubes in each bowl and transfer the eggs with a slotted spoon to the bowls. Sprinkle the eggs and soup with salt and serve.

MAKE 4 SERVINGS.

--- NUTRIENT ANALYSIS PER SERVING: ---

Calories (kcal) 298 ■ Protein (g) 10.6 ■ Carbohydrates (g) 20 ■ Fat (g) 20 ■ Saturated Fat (g) 3.7 ■ Sodium (mg) 342 ■ Cholesterol (mg) 212.5 ■ % Calories from Protein 14 ■ % Calories from Carbohydrates 27 ■ % Calories from Fat 61 ■ Total Dietary Fiber (g) 2.9

POTATO AND SPINACH SOUP

T HIS SOUP, THOUGH comforting, is very flavorful, unlike the bland, tasteless soups people with GERD think they're doomed to eat. The onion in this recipe is an important flavor booster, though the amount has been reduced significantly from the original recipe. This is a great use for leftover mashed potatoes, but, if the leftover potatoes are seasoned, be sure not to add too much salt to the soup.

> 2 tablespoons olive oil
> ½ cup minced onion (as tolerated)
> 3 cups mashed potatoes
> 6 cups fat-free chicken broth, water, or vegetable broth
> ½ teaspoon ground nutmeg
> 1 (10-ounce) package frozen leaf spinach, thawed
> Salt to taste
> Grated fresh Parmesan cheese, garnish (optional)

1. Heat oil in a large sauce pan or soup pot over medium high heat. Add the onions, if using, and sauté for 3 minutes.
2. Add the mashed potatoes and stir well. Add the broth and nutmeg and stir until smooth.
3. Bring the soup to a boil, reduce heat, and cook for 15 minutes, stirring occasionally.
4. Stir in the spinach and cook for 5 minutes more. Season to taste with salt and serve with grated Parmesan cheese, if desired.

MAKES 8 SERVINGS.

NUTRIENT ANALYSIS PER SERVING:

Calories (kcal) 175 ■ Protein (g) 4 ■ Carbohydrates (g) 20 ■ Fat (g) 9.5 ■ Saturated Fat (g) 2 ■ Sodium (mg) 452 ■ Cholesterol (mg) 3.4 ■ % Calories from Protein 9 ■ % Calories from Carbohydrates 45 ■ % Calories from Fat 49 ■ Total Dietary Fiber (g) 3.5

Lentil Soup

Lentils, like beans, are full of protein and naturally fat-free. Lentil soup is often included as part of the Mediterranean diet so popular these days. Lentils take longer than other foods for the body to digest, so you feel full longer. This recipe doesn't specify which type of lentils to use, so try red or green for variety.

> 2 tablespoons olive oil
> 1 cup diced carrots
> ½ cup diced celery
> 8 cups water or vegetable broth
> 2 cups dry lentils, rinsed
> ½ teaspoon ground cumin
> ½ cup fresh chopped parsley
> Salt to taste

1. Combine all ingredients except salt in a large pot over medium-high heat and bring to a boil.
2. Reduce heat, and cook the soup for 40 minutes to an hour, until the lentils are softened and the soup is thick (you may need to add more liquid if the broth evaporates too quickly—keep adding just enough to make the soup "soupy").
3. Add salt to taste and serve hot.

Makes 6–8 servings.

Nutrient Analysis Per Serving:

Calories (kcal) 269 ■ Protein (g) 18.4 ■ Carbohydrates (g) 39 ■ Fat (g) 5.2 ■ Saturated Fat (g) .7 ■ Sodium (mg) 122 ■ Cholesterol (mg) 0 ■ % Calories from Protein 27 ■ % Calories from Carbohydrates 59 ■ % Calories from Fat 18 ■ Total Dietary Fiber (g) 20.5

CHUNKY CORN CHOWDER

THICK AND HEARTY, this corn chowder will keep you warm all day long, but won't give you reflux. Onion, omnipresent in most chowders, has been reduced significantly, and fat is very low. If you have a problem with dairy products, substitute nondairy creamer for the evaporated milk.

> 4 tablespoons extra virgin olive oil
> ½ cup onion, chopped (as tolerated)
> 1 cup diced red bell pepper
> 1 cup diced green bell pepper
> 1 cup chopped celery
> ½ tablespoon ground nutmeg
> ½ cup all-purpose flour
> 2 cups fat-free chicken broth or water
> 2 cups fat-free evaporated milk
> 4 cups fresh or frozen corn kernels, thawed
> Kosher salt to taste

1. Heat oil in a large saucepan over medium-high heat.
2. Add onion, bell peppers, and celery and cook for 5 minutes, until the vegetables are softened.
3. Add the nutmeg and flour and cook, stirring for 3 minutes more.
4. Add the broth and milk and bring mixture to boil, whisking to remove lumps and mix through.
5. Stir in the corn and bring the mixture to a boil. Reduce the heat and cook for 10 minutes more, adding more liquids as needed. Add salt to taste and serve hot.

MAKES 8 SERVINGS.

NUTRIENT ANALYSIS PER SERVING:

Calories (kcal) 227 ■ Protein (g) 8.7 ■ Carbohydrates (g) 34 ■ Fat (g) 7.7 ■ Saturated Fat (g) 1 ■ Sodium (mg) 134 ■ Cholesterol (mg) 2.3 ■ % Calories from Protein 15 ■ % Calories from Carbohydrates 60 ■ % Calories from Fat 31 ■ Total Dietary Fiber (g) 3

Salad Days

WHILE IN THE past Americans thought of salad as merely a segue to the entrée, it's no longer fashionable to assume it's just a fresh beginning of a great meal, but rather to see it as *the* meal itself. Heavy—fattening and reflux inciting—foods get shoved to the back of the fridge or packed away and frozen, as we make room for everything from the garden. The salad spinner finds a permanent, accessible spot on our kitchen counter because it's elevated to the most useful tool in the kitchen.

Salads are a nearly perfect meal choice for folks with GERD. They're often low in calories (if you leave the fattening dressings to a minimum), and filling, and they satisfy the craving for chewy foods. And the added fiber in vegetables makes them quicker to digest.

Greens—leafy, sweet, bitter, chewy and buttery—are often the substructure of what we think of as salad. The cucumbers, carrots, et al, are the ornamentation, necessary because they are what attract us—visually and tastily—with fork in hand to stab at our meals. Some of the recipes here include bell peppers as an ingredient. While hot peppers and chilis contain varying amounts of capsaicin, an oily substance that gives peppers their scorching attributes and universally causes discomfort, sweet bell peppers are tolerable for almost everybody.

If adding meats, fowl, or fish to a salad will make it seem heartier, do it, by all means. Cheese and beans will add yet more protein, though they must be consumed with caution. Portion control is important here. Large quantities of fatty cheese and meat can add to calorie counts, which lead to weight gain and a potentially weakened LES.

The best dressed salads for those with reflux are those which are not very spicy or overdressed with higher-fat oils, large amounts of acidic vinegar, or citrus. As stated earlier in the book, there are a couple of ways to relieve the acid in vinegar: use less vinegar or use vinegar with lower acidity. Vinegar is made with various acidity levels, the percentage of which is listed on product labels. For example, one balsamic vinegar may register 6 percent acidity while a white wine vinegar may register 5 percent, so switching to lower acidity vinegar is an option.

The salads below are lightly dressed, a concept that will take some getting used to for many folks. What you're left with is the true flavors of the foods you're eating.

Green Beans with Pecans and Warm Honeyed Apple Dressing

Green beans offer high fiber and low calories. Pecans are high in fat, but, used sparingly, are also an additional good source of fiber, as are the apples. This is a great side dish to serve with just about any meal, especially if the entrée is more plain than fancy. The apples give these beans an autumn bent, but they're great any time of the year. Substitute pears for the apple, for a completely different flavor.

    2 pounds green beans
    2 cups chopped Granny Smith apples
    ¼ cup olive oil
    1 teaspoon fresh minced garlic (as tolerated)
    3 tablespoons honey
    2 tablespoons balsamic vinegar (as tolerated)
    ¼ cup apple cider
    1 tablespoon grainy or Dijon mustard (as tolerated)
    ¼ cup crumbed blue cheese, any type, or feta cheese, any type
        (as tolerated)
    ¼ cup chopped pecans, lightly toasted

1. Trim the stem ends from rinsed green beans (leave the pointed ends untouched).
2. Bring a pot of water to a boil and drop in the green beans. Blanche the beans until bright green, about 1 minute. Drain the beans, rinse them under cold water, and drain well.
3. Meanwhile, combine the apples, oil, garlic, honey, vinegar, cider, and mustard in a small saucepan over medium-high heat and bring to a boil. Remove from heat and cool until warm.
4. Arrange the green beans on a platter. Sprinkle blue cheese, if using, over the beans. Sprinkle the pecans over the beans.
5. Stir the warm dressing well and spoon it over the beans.

Makes 8 servings.

Nutrient Analysis Per Serving:

Calories (kcal) 180 ■ Protein (g) 3.2 ■ Carbohydrates (g) 21 ■ Fat (g) 10.6 ■ Saturated Fat (g) 2 ■ Sodium (mg) 92 ■ Cholesterol (mg) 3 ■ % Calories from Protein 7 ■ % Calories from Carbohydrates 46 ■ % Calories from Fat 53 ■ Total Dietary Fiber (g) 4.5

SALADE NICOISE WITH SEARED AHI TUNA

SALADE NICOISE IS the signature salad from the south of France. Eaten as a meal, rather than just a side dish, this variation of the famous French salad uses fresh tuna instead of the canned variety. Gone are onions and most of the garlic, two major triggers. And because the salad is light, you won't feel overly full. This recipe calls for a small amount of fresh lemon juice. If this is a trigger for you, leave it out. The results will still be very good. If you're strapped for time, use canned tuna to make this salad, as they do in France. Just skip the marinating and searing and go straight for the assembly. Remember to use less canned tuna; you won't need as much.

DRESSING:

  ½ cup extra virgin olive oil or canola oil
  2 tablespoons red wine vinegar
  Juice of 1 lemon (as tolerated)
  1 teaspoon fresh minced garlic (as tolerated)
  1 teaspoon dried tarragon
  2 tablspoons drained capers
  Salt to taste

SALAD:

  2 pounds Ahi tuna, cut into 6 steaks
  12 red skin potatoes, quartered
  4 ripe tomatoes, cut into wedges (as tolerated)
  6 chopped hardboiled egg whites
  ½ cup black or Niçoise olives
  1 can (about 15 ounces) great northern beans, rinsed and drained
  1 pound green beans
  1 tablespoon drained capers
  1 cup chopped parsley
  1 small can flat anchovies, drained

1. Make dressing: combine all dressing ingredients in a small bowl and whisk well. Set aside.
2. Arrange tuna in a shallow dish. Pour ¼ of the vinaigrette over the fish. Cover with plastic wrap, chill, and marinate for 2 hours, turning once or twice during the marinating.

3. Make salad: Bring a large pot of water to a boil over high heat. Add the potatoes and cook until al dente, about 25 minutes. Using a large slotted spoon, remove the potatoes to a colander, rinse under cold water, and drain very well. Divide the potatoes among 6 dinner-sized plates.

4. Bring the water to a boil again and blanche the green beans until al dente, about one minute. Drain and rinse with cold water.

5. Divide and arrange the green beans, great northern beans, tomatoes, egg whites, and olives on the plates next to the potatoes, in sections (do not toss the salad).

6. Heat a heavy large skillet over high heat—the skillet must be very hot. Spray the fish on both sides with nonstick cooking spray. Carefully place tuna steaks in the skillet (you may need to do this in 2 skillets to accommodate the tuna, or cook the tuna in batches). Brown on all sides, turning occasionally, about 10–12 minutes total, for medium-rare tuna. Transfer the tuna to the salad, placing the steak on top of the other vegetables or next to them.

7. Whisk the remaining dressing again before drizzling it over the entire salad. Garnish the salad with the anchovies and capers; sprinkle with the chopped parsley. Serve immediately for hot tuna or serve the salad at room temperature.

MAKES 6 SERVINGS.

NUTRIENT ANALYSIS PER SERVING:

Calories (kcal) 480 ∎ Protein (g) 41 ∎ Carbohydrates (g) 30 ∎ Fat (g) 22 ∎ Saturated Fat (g) 3 ∎ Sodium (mg) 898 ∎ Cholesterol (mg) 61.6 ∎ % Calories from Protein 34 ∎ % Calories from Carbohydrates 25 ∎ % Calories from Fat 42 ∎ Total Dietary Fiber (g) 8.3

RED CABBAGE SLAW
WITH CREAMY POPPY SEED DRESSING

C ABBAGE IS ONE of those "gassy" vegetables. However, much of the gas that is produced from these vegetables is produced by the bacteria in the colon, the location of which rules out the notion that the gas will migrate back to the stomach and place pressure on the LES. This creamy slaw tastes as good as more fat-filled versions. The red cabbage will turn the dressing pink. If you like your slaw a more "usual" color, switch to green cabbage. And if you prefer your salad less dressed, use less dressing or more cabbage. It's an easily modified recipe.

> 6 cups finely shredded red cabbage
> 2 cups shredded carrots
> 1 cup chopped scallions, white and green parts (as tolerated)

DRESSING:

> $\frac{1}{2}$ cup fat-free mayonnaise
> $\frac{1}{2}$ cup fat-free sour cream
> $\frac{1}{3}$ cup honey
> 2 tablespoons poppy seeds
> 1 tablespoon Dijon mustard (as tolerated)
> Juice of l lemon, about $\frac{1}{4}$ cup (as tolerated)
> Salt to taste

1. Place cabbage, carrots, and scallions (if using), in a large bowl and toss to combine. Set aside.
2. In a separate bowl, combine all dressing ingredients and whisk well to combine.
3. Pour half this dressing over the cabbage mixture and toss well, adding more if needed, to desired consistency.

MAKES 8 SERVINGS.

NUTRIENT ANALYSIS PER SERVING:

Calories (kcal) 115 ■ Protein (g) 2.8 ■ Carbohydrates (g) 24.6 ■ Fat (g) 1.2 ■ Saturated Fat (g) 0 ■ Sodium (mg) 179 ■ Cholesterol (mg) 0 ■ % Calories from Protein 10 ■ % Calories from Carbohydrates 86 ■ % Calories from Fat 10 ■ Total Dietary Fiber (g) 2.5

ASPARAGUS AND ARTICHOKE SALAD WITH ASIAGO AND BASIL

ASPARAGUS IS NATURALLY lean, so the small amount of fat from the olive oil and Asiago cheese make this dish appropriate occasionally. The recipe instructs you to peel thick asparagus stalks. Look for thin stalks to avoid this step. The amount of water called for in this recipe steams the asparagus instead of boiling it, ensuring bright green stalks and a crisp-tender crunch.

2 pounds fresh asparagus, trimmed and peeled if the stalks are thick
1 red bell pepper, sliced into very thin strips
1 cup water
1 can (about 15 ounces) quartered artichoke hearts, drained
1/2 teaspoon dried oregano
Kosher salt to taste
1/2 cup grated or shredded Asiago cheese (as tolerated)
1/2 cup fresh basil leaves, whole
3 tablespoons extra virgin olive oil
2 tablespoons balsamic vinegar (as tolerated)

1. Heat asparagus and red pepper with one cup of water in a large covered pot over high heat. When the water boils, turn off the heat and let the vegetables steam for about 5 minutes more. Remove the vegetables to a colander, rinse with cold water, and drain well.
2. Arrange the asparagus and peppers on a platter. Arrange the artichoke hearts over and around the asparagus. Sprinkle the oregano and kosher salt over. Sprinkle cheese over all and garnish with the basil leaves.
3. Drizzle olive oil and vinegar over and serve.

MAKES 6 SERVINGS.

NUTRIENT ANALYSIS PER SERVING:

Calories (kcal) 185 ■ Protein (g) 10 ■ Carbohydrates (g) 8 ■ Fat (g) 12 ■ Saturated Fat (g) 4.3 ■ Sodium (mg) 361 ■ Cholesterol (mg) 16.7 ■ % Calories from Protein 21 ■ % Calories from Carbohydrates 17 ■ % Calories from Fat 59 ■ Total Dietary Fiber (g) 1.7

ROMAINE SALAD WITH TUNA, WHITE BEANS, AND GREEK OLIVES

THE INGREDIENTS IN this Mediterranean salad pack a powerful nutritional punch. A cousin to the similar Salade Nicoise, the lettuce adds fiber, and the tuna and beans add texture and even more protein to this super-healthy salad. The dressing has lowered amounts of vinegar and mustard and just a small amount of oregano for flavor.

> 2 red bell peppers
> 4 hearts of romaine lettuce, separated into leaves, uncut
> 4 cans (6.5 ounces each) Albacore white tuna in water, drained
> 1 can (about 15 ounces), great northern beans, drained well
> 32 Kalamata or other Greek olives
> 2 tablespoons drained capers
> ½ cup fresh chopped parsley
> 16 anchovy fillets (as tolerated)

DRESSING:
> ⅓ cup extra-virgin olive oil
> 1 tablespoon Dijon mustard
> 2 tablespoons fresh chopped oregano (or ½ tsp. dry)
> Kosher salt to taste
> Lemon wedges, optional

1. Roast peppers: Preheat broiler. Place peppers directly on an upper rack of the oven (about 6 inches from the top) with a cookie sheet on the rack just below to capture juices. Roast the peppers, turning them with tongs, until skins are blackened all around, about 10 minutes or more. Remove them from the oven and wrap them in foil to cool for at least 10 minutes. Scrape away and remove most of the peppers' peel with your hands, remove seeds, and cut the peppers into thin strips. Set aside.
2. Make dressing: Combine all dressing ingredients in a medium bowl and whisk well. Set aside.
3. Arrange salad: Arrange uncut romaine leaves on 8 individual dinner plates. Set aside.
4. Place tuna in a medium bowl and gently break into pieces (do not mash). Arrange the tuna over the core-end (whiter part) of the romaine leaves.

5. Sprinkle beans over the tuna and lettuce. Arrange the olives around the plate and sprinkle the capers over all.
6. Carefully spoon the dressing over the salad and sprinkle parsley over all.
7. Arrange two anchovies over the salad, if using. Serve with lemon wedges, if using.

MAKES 8 SERVINGS.

NUTRIENT ANALYSIS PER SERVING:

Calories (kcal) 282 ■ Protein (g) 26 ■ Carbohydrates (g) 11.6 ■ Fat (g) 14.6 ■ Saturated Fat (g) 2.3 ■ Sodium (mg) 1,008 ■ Cholesterol (mg) 42.5 ■ % Calories from Protein 37 ■ % Calories from Carbohydrates 16 ■ % Calories from Fat 47 ■ Total Dietary Fiber (g) 4.6

SHRIMP AND PAPAYA SALAD

VERY LOW IN fat and with easily tolerated papaya and cilantro, this salad seems like an unusual combination. But only here in the United States. In the tropics, this is a natural combination that's both sweet and tart. The amount of acid has been reduced in the light dressing, and calories from added oil are also reduced.

> *1 pound large shrimp, shelled (25–30 per pound)*
> *2 cups ¼-inch diced papaya*
> *⅓ cup fresh cilantro, chopped*
> *½ cup shredded carrots*
> *1 cup chopped scallions (as tolerated)*
> *8 cups chopped romaine lettuce*
> *2 cups fresh bean sprouts*
> *¼ cup extra virgin olive oil*
> *¼ cup orange juice, low acid if possible (as tolerated)*
> *Kosher salt to taste*

1. Bring a medium pot of water to a boil over high heat. Add shrimp and cook for about one minute, until just cooked through (do not overcook or the shrimp will be rubbery). Transfer the shrimp to a colander, drain, and rinse under cold water to stop cooking. Halve shrimp vertically and devein.
2. Toss shrimp, papaya, cilantro, carrot, and scallions, if using, in a large bowl to combine.
3. Divide the lettuce among 8 salad plates. Sprinkle bean sprouts over them. Divide the shrimp and papaya mixture over the salads. Set aside.
4. Combine the olive oil and orange juice in a small bowl and whisk well. Drizzle this dressing over the salad. Sprinkle the salads with salt and serve.

MAKES 8 SERVINGS.

NUTRIENT ANALYSIS PER SERVING:

Calories (kcal) 156 ■ Protein (g) 14 ■ Carbohydrates (g) 9 ■ Fat (g) 7.6 ■ Saturated Fat (g) 1 ■ Sodium (mg) 149 ■ Cholesterol (mg) 110 ■ % Calories from Protein 36 ■ % Calories from Carbohydrates 23 ■ % Calories from Fat 44 ■ Total Dietary Fiber (g) 2.7

Napa Salad with Mango, Papaya, and Jicama

THIS SALAD OF gentle mango and papaya is noisy to eat. The soft cabbage, though often gas producing, should not be bothersome, as much of the gas produced by any cabbage is produced by bacteria in the colon. As stated earlier in the book, the location means it's unlikely gas will migrate back to the stomach and place pressure on the LES. Jicama has the texture of apples, so it's crunchy and filling. The tropical fruit adds sweetness. The dressing is sweet and sour, good enough to use as a marinade or simply tossed with fresh fruit to serve at your brunch table.

DRESSING:

    1 tablespoon sugar
    2 tablespoons red-wine vinegar (as tolerated)
    2 tablespoons apple cider or juice
    1 tablespoon minced gingerroot
    ¼ cup light olive oil
    2 tablespoons light soy sauce
    1 tablespoon sesame seeds

SALAD:

    2 cups peeled jicama, cut into thin slices
    2 mangoes, peeled and diced
    2 cups diced papaya
    4 cups shredded napa cabbage
    2 cups diced seeded cucumber
    ¼ cup slivered almonds, lightly toasted
    1 cup chopped scallions, white and green parts (as tolerated)

1. Make dressing: Combine all ingredients in a small bowl and whisk to combine. Set aside.
2. Make salad: Toss all salad ingredients in a large bowl with the dressing.

MAKES 8 SERVINGS.

NUTRIENT ANALYSIS PER SERVING:

Calories (kcal) 177 ■ Protein (g) 3 ■ Carbohydrates (g) 22 ■ Fat (g) 10 ■ Saturated Fat (g) 1.2 ■ Sodium (mg) 146 ■ Cholesterol (mg) 0 ■ % Calories from Protein 7 ■ % Calories from Carbohydrates 49 ■ % Calories from Fat 50 ■ Total Dietary Fiber (g) 5.5

WHEAT BERRY SALAD
WITH GRILLED CHICKEN AND PEAS

THIS FILLING SALAD is very low in fat and full of fiber and protein. Wheat berries are chewy, with the texture of al dente barley. They're whole berries of wheat, unprocessed, and eaten like rice. In fact, you may substitute brown or wild rice for the wheat berries in this recipe.

> *2 cups wheat berries*
> *6 cups water or vegetable broth*
> *1 pound boneless and skinless chicken breasts, trimmed of visible fat*
> *3 tablespoons olive oil*
> *1 cup fresh cooked or frozen peas, defrosted*
> *1 cup diced carrots*
> *1 cup diced seedless cucumber*
> *1 cup chopped celery*
> *1 cup fresh chopped parsley*
> *Salt to taste*
> *12 cups mixed baby or field greens*
> *¼–½ cup balsamic vinegar (as tolerated)*
> *½ cup olive oil*

1. Combine wheat berries and water in a saucepan over medium-high heat. Bring the water to a boil, reduce heat, and simmer the wheat berries for an hour, covered, until tender. Drain, rinse under cold water, and drain well.
2. While the wheat berries are cooking, brush the chicken breasts with olive oil and grill over medium-high heat or broil until just cooked through. Allow the chicken to cool slightly before cutting it into 1-inch chunks.
3. Place the cooked, drained wheat berries in a large bowl. Add the cooled chicken, peas, carrots, cucumber, celery, and parsley and toss well. Season to taste with salt.
4. Arrange the greens on 8 individual plates and divide the wheat berry mixture over. Serve with balsamic vinegar and olive oil on the side or drizzle the vinegar and oil over each salad to taste.

MAKES 8 SERVINGS.

--- **NUTRIENT ANALYSIS PER SERVING:** ---

Calories (kcal) 445 ■ Protein (g) 23 ■ Carbohydrates (g) 44 ■ Fat (g) 21.4 ■ Saturated Fat (g) 3 ■ Sodium (mg) 118 ■ Cholesterol (mg) 34.7 ■ % Calories from Protein 20 ■ % Calories from Carbohydrates 39 ■ % Calories from Fat 43 ■ Total Dietary Fiber (g) 9.3

Tabouli Pasta Salad

Pasta salad can be very caloric. It's often not good for those trying to keep weight down to control GERD. This enlightened salad borrows flavors from the Middle Eastern tabouli salad normally made with cracked wheat called bulgur. There are small amounts of raw chopped onion and garlic in this recipe—tolerable for some, dynamite for others. If you're very sensitive, eat this salad no later than at lunch, or leave the offending ingredients out. For variety, or to make this more of an entrée, add four cups of cubed, grilled chicken breast to the mix.

> 3 cups fresh minced parsley
> ½ cup fresh chopped dill
> 1 cup diced cucumber
> 1 cup seeded, diced tomato (as tolerated), or 1½ cups ½-inch diced zucchini
> ¼ cup chopped red or Bermuda onion (as tolerated)
> 1 teaspoon minced garlic (as tolerated)
> 3 tablespoons light soy sauce
> ¼ cup extra virgin olive oil
> Kosher salt to taste
> ½ pound or more dry penne or other shaped pasta, cooked al dente, according to package directions, drained, rinsed under cold water, and drained well again.

1. Combine parsley, dill, cucumber, tomato, onion, garlic, soy sauce, and olive oil in a large bowl and toss well.
2. Add the pasta and toss well.
3. Add salt to taste. Serve at room temperature.

Makes 12 side dish servings.

Nutrient Analysis Per Serving:

Calories (kcal) 125 ▪ Protein (g) 3.5 ▪ Carbohydrates (g) 16.9 ▪ Fat (g) 5 ▪ Saturated Fat (g) 0 ▪ Sodium (mg) 159 ▪ Cholesterol (mg) 0 ▪ % Calories from Protein 11 ▪ % Calories from Carbohydrates 54 ▪ % Calories from Fat 36 ▪ Total Dietary Fiber (g) 1.3

Broiled Pear and Endive Salad with Corn and Caper Vinaigrette

THIS SALAD IS dressy with its lovely arranged—and low acid—pears combined with the bitter Belgian endive. The dressing is very light, relying on the corn, cheese, and crunchy nuts to add more flavor. And the combination of sweet and bitter is very engaging.

SALAD:

3 heads Belgian endive

3 ripe pears (any variety), unpeeled and cut into thin wedges

1 tablespoon olive oil

1 cup fresh raw or frozen corn kernels, thawed

½ cup crumbled Gorgonzola cheese (as tolerated)

¼ cup pine nuts, lightly toasted

½ cup fresh chopped parsley

Kosher salt to taste

VINAIGRETTE:

1 tablespoon olive oil

1 tablespoon walnut oil

1 tablespoon red wine vinegar (as tolerated)

2 teaspoons Dijon mustard (as tolerated)

1 tablespoon drained capers

2–3 tablespoons fresh chopped dill

1. Cut the bottoms off the endive and arrange the spears on a small serving platter in a sunburst pattern (points pointed out).
2. Preheat oven to broil. Arrange pear slices on a baking sheet that's been sprayed with nonstick cooking spray. Drizzle the pears with the olive oil. Place the baking sheet in the top third of the oven. Broil the pears with the oven door slightly open until lightly colored. Remove the pears from the oven and let cool. Arrange the cooled pear slices on the platter, overlapping the endives slightly.
3. Sprinkle salad with corn, cheese, pine nuts, and parsley.

4. Combine all the vinaigrette ingredients in a small bowl and whisk well. Drizzle the vinaigrette over the salad. Sprinkle the salad with salt to taste and serve.

MAKES 6 SERVINGS.

——— NUTRIENT ANALYSIS PER SERVING: ———

Calories (kcal) 214 ■ Protein (g) 5.4 ■ Carbohydrates (g) 21 ■ Fat (g) 13.6 ■ Saturated Fat (g) 3.4 ■ Sodium (mg) 247 ■ Cholesterol (mg) 8.5 ■ % Calories from Protein 10 ■ % Calories from Carbohydrates 39 ■ % Calories from Fat 57 ■ Total Dietary Fiber (g) 3.8

Spinach and Watercress Salad with Peaches and Warm Herb Dressing

SPINACH SALADS ARE often served with fatty bacon, acidic orange slices, and loads of oily dressing, all of which can trigger bouts of GERD. This recipe retains the flavor of traditional spinach salads, with the sweetness coming from soothing peaches instead of oranges. And because the dressing greatly reduces the normal amounts of oil and vinegar, and contains just a small amount of shallots, it's also much less offensive. If the mere idea of shallots is bothersome, however, leave them out entirely.

This salad also uses baby spinach, which often comes prewashed and ready to eat. It's much more delicate and less chewy than the large, curly spinach you may be used to. The warm dressing "wilts" the spinach slightly, giving it a silky texture. For more variety, add chopped egg whites, dried fruits, even chickpeas, to the salad if desired.

DRESSING:

⅓ cup olive oil
⅓ cup finely chopped shallots (as tolerated)
2 tablespoons red wine vinegar (as tolerated)
2 tablespoons fresh tarragon leaves or 1 teaspoon dried
2 tablespoons fresh basil leaves, chopped, or 1 teaspoon dried
1 teaspoon kosher salt

SALAD:

12–14 cups fresh baby spinach leaves, thick stems trimmed
1 large bunch watercress, thick stems trimmed
2 peaches, unpeeled, cut into thin wedges
½ cup chopped pecans, lightly toasted

1. Make dressing: Heat oil in medium saucepan over medium-low heat. Add shallots and sauté until softened, about 4 minutes. Allow to cool slightly before stirring in remaining ingredients. Set aside.
2. Make salad: Toss spinach and watercress in a large bowl. Set aside.
3. Heat dressing over medium-high heat until hot and toss with the salad.
4. Quickly divide the salad among 8 large salad or dinner plates.

5. Divide peach slices among the salads, sprinkle with the chopped pecans, and serve.

MAKES 8 SERVINGS.

NUTRIENT ANALYSIS PER SERVING:

Calories (kcal) 136 ■ Protein (g) 2.3 ■ Carbohydrates (g) 2.6 ■ Fat (g) 13.6 ■ Saturated Fat (g) 1.6 ■ Sodium (mg) 283 ■ Cholesterol (mg) 0 ■ % Calories from Protein 7 ■ % Calories from Carbohydrates 8 ■ % Calories from Fat 90 ■ Total Dietary Fiber (g) 5.2

Mom's Potato Salad

Ordinary potato salads are mostly creamy. That translates into heavy, fatty dressings. Some also contain big chunks of egg, which also adds to calories. This doesn't mean you have to give up potato salad altogether. This potato salad makeover is a crowd-pleaser because it's still creamy, using nonfat mayonnaise instead of the high-fat version, lean egg whites, and a surprise ingredient—capers. Remember, the small amount of vinegar and mustard is distributed throughout this large salad.

> 3 pounds peeled russet or Idaho potatoes cut into 1-inch chunks
> ¼ cup red wine vinegar (as tolerated)
> ½–1 cup nonfat mayonnaise
> 1 tablespoon Dijon mustard (as tolerated)
> 12 hard-boiled egg whites, chopped
> 1 cup chopped celery
> ¼ cup sweet pickle relish (as tolerated)
> Kosher salt to taste
> 1 cup frozen peas, thawed
> 1 cup ¼-inch diced carrots, steamed or cooked lightly
> 3 tablespoons dried parsley flakes
> 1 tablespoon drained capers
> Paprika and chopped fresh parsley, garnish

1. Place potatoes in a large pot of cold water over high heat. Bring the water to a boil, reduce heat slightly, and boil potatoes for 12–15 minutes until just tender.
2. Remove from heat and drain the potatoes well (do not rinse), shaking colander to remove all excess water.
3. Place the hot, drained potatoes in a large bowl and sprinkle them with the vinegar, if using. Allow the potatoes to cool to room temperature.
4. Add the mayonnaise, beginning with ½-cup, and mustard, and toss well. Fold in the egg, celery, relish, and salt.
5. Add more mayonnaise until the salad is to your desired creaminess. Fold in the peas, carrots, dried parsley, and capers.
6. Arrange the potato salad on a platter or in a serving bowl, cover, and chill until ready to serve.

7. Garnish with parsley and sprinkle with paprika just before serving.

Makes 12 or more servings.

Nutrient Analysis Per Serving:

Calories (kcal) 117 ■ Protein (g) 6.7 ■ Carbohydrates (g) 21 ■ Fat (g) 0.3 ■ Saturated Fat (g) 0 ■ Sodium (mg) 323 ■ Cholesterol (mg) 0 ■ % Calories from Protein 23 ■ % Calories from Carbohydrates 72 ■ % Calories from Fat 3 ■ Total Dietary Fiber (g) 2.7

Mixed Greens Salad with Smoked Salmon Rose and Tarragon Vinaigrette

COLD SMOKED SALMON, such as lox, is the centerpiece of this unusually beautiful entrée salad. The salad itself is completely GERD-friendly. The dressing is very light, yet flavorful, cutting offensive ingredients to a minimum. If desired make the salad smaller and serve it as a first course. Edible flower petals should be organically grown and free of pesticides. Look for them at specialty food stores or at farmers' markets.

SALAD:

    16 cups mixed salad greens, of any type
    ½ cup fresh chopped dill
    ½ cup assorted edible flower petals, such as nasturtium, roses, marigolds, dandelions, chive flowers, and pansies; wash gently, optional (as tolerated)
    1 cup ½-inch diced, peeled, seeded cucumber
    ¼ cup sunflower seeds
    32 very thin slices of smoked salmon or lox (each slice about the same size) (about 1 ounce)

DRESSING:

    2 tablespoons red wine or balsamic vinegar (as tolerated)
    1–2 tablespoons orange blossom or flower water, or to taste (available at specialty food shops)
    ¼ cup extra virgin olive oil
    1 teaspoon sugar
    1 tablespoon fresh tarragon, minced, or ½ tsp. dried
    Kosher salt to taste

1. Toss the greens and fresh dill in a large bowl. Arrange the greens on individual dinner-sized plates.
2. Sprinkle the flower petals over the greens, if using.
3. Sprinkle the cucumber and sunflower seeds over all.
4. Make salmon roses: Roll 1 thin slice of salmon loosely into a "tube." Wrap another slice loosely around the first slice and continue with 2 more slices until the rolls form a loose flower rose. "Fluff" or arrange the salmon "petals." Flatten the

bottom of the "salmon rose" with your hand so that it can sit squarely on the greens. Transfer the rose to the center of a salad. Repeat with remaining salmon. Set aside.

5. Make dressing: Combine all dressing ingredients in a bowl and whisk until smooth. Drizzle the dressing over the salads and serve.

MAKES 8 SERVINGS.

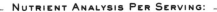

NUTRIENT ANALYSIS PER SERVING:

Calories (kcal) 173 ■ Protein (g) 13 ■ Carbohydrates (g) 4.6 ■ Fat (g) 11.6 ■ Saturated Fat (g) 1.7 ■ Sodium (mg) 1,144 ■ Cholesterol (mg) 13 ■ % Calories from Protein 31 ■ % Calories from Carbohydrates 11 ■ % Calories from Fat 61 ■ Total Dietary Fiber (g) 2.5

SIDESHOW

SIDE DISHES ARE the supporting players of every meal. They're especially important for those with GERD, since day-to-day entrees tend to be simple and unadorned—grilled fish or chicken, often minimally seasoned.

They're also important because they serve to balance the entrée and add visual appeal to the plate. Mom's old rule of "something green" can be any color of the vegetable rainbow, and starches have come a long way from rice and baked potatoes.

The good news is that of all the meal components, the choices for side dishes are virtually endless. Most foods, except those we know are triggers, are permissible. Most sides, in general, contain negligible amounts of citrus, vinegar, sugar, chocolate, peppermint, caffeine, or alcohol. Hot peppers and pepper sauces are often easily reduced or eliminated altogether from most recipes, as these are often condiments rather than main ingredients.

Dairy, an exception, is often listed among ingredients for creamy pastas, grains, and pureed potatoes, and is available in less-offensive low-and no-fat versions as well as in substitute versions made with soy. Fresh herbs and their dried counterparts are more available in well-stocked markets, and the variety of available vegetables, pastas, and grains is extensive.

Go ahead and eat those sides, in moderation, of course. After all, what you serve alongside your main dish should be as interesting at the main course itself. Look to balance flavors, colors, and textures when you serve these or any of your favorite sides. Of course there's still nothing wrong with a baked potato; just don't overstuff it with butter, fatty meats, or cheeses, which add calories quickly.

HERB AND OLIVE OIL ROASTED GREEN BEANS

Roasting vegetables gives them completely different flavors and textures from boiled or steamed vegetables. They seem earthy and filling. While this recipe calls for green beans, feel free to substitute any of your favorite vegetables. Keep in mind that cooking times may vary for different vegetables.

> *2 pounds green beans*
> *2 tablespoons olive oil*
> *1 tablespoon fresh rosemary or ½ teaspoon dried rosemary*
> *1 tablespoon fresh dill or ½ teaspoon dried dill*
> *1 tablespoon fresh oregano or ½ teaspoon dried oregano*
> *Kosher salt to taste*

1. Preheat oven to 400° F.
2. Trim the stem ends from rinsed green beans (leave the pointed ends untouched).
3. Toss beans with oil and herbs in a bowl and transfer them to a large, shallow baking pan or dish.
4. Roast uncovered for 20 minutes.
5. Remove from oven and sprinkle with salt, to taste. Toss the beans to distribute the salt. Serve the beans hot or at room temperature.

Makes 8 servings.

NUTRIENT ANALYSIS PER SERVING:

Calories (kcal) 66 ■ Protein (g) 2 ■ Carbohydrates (g) 8 ■ Fat (g) 3.5 ■ Saturated Fat (g) 0.5 ■ Sodium (mg) 42 ■ Cholesterol (mg) 0 ■ % Calories from Protein 13 ■ % Calories from Carbohydrates 50 ■ % Calories from Fat 48 ■ Total Dietary Fiber (g) 4

BRAISED SPINACH WITH PINE NUTS

A SMALL AMOUNT of garlic is called for in this quick-and-easy recipe—just enough to flavor the oil slightly, for the three pounds of spinach you're using. Pine nuts add texture and flavor, with very little fat. For variety, use almonds, pistachios, or chopped walnuts instead of the pine nuts.

3 pounds baby spinach
3 tablespoons olive oil
$\frac{1}{2}$ teaspoon garlic (as tolerated)
$\frac{1}{4}$ cup pine nuts, lightly toasted
Kosher salt to taste

1. Rinse spinach well, if needed, and remove any unusually large stems. Set aside.
2. Heat oil and garlic, if using, in a large nonstick skillet over medium-high heat, and cook, stirring for 1 minute.
3. Add spinach (in batches if you must) and cook, turning the leaves frequently with tongs, until just wilted. Stir in pine nuts.
4. Remove from heat and transfer the spinach to a serving dish. Sprinkle salt over the spinach to taste. Serve hot or warm.

MAKES 8 SERVINGS.

NUTRIENT ANALYSIS PER SERVING:

Calories (kcal) 115 ■ Protein (g) 7.7 ■ Carbohydrates (g) 1.3 ■ Fat (g) 10.3 ■ Saturated Fat (g) 1.3 ■ Sodium (mg) 293 ■ Cholesterol (mg) 0 ■ % Calories from Protein 27 ■ % Calories from Carbohydrates 5 ■ % Calories from Fat 81 ■ Total Dietary Fiber (g) 20

SHORTCUT SESAME PEAS AND SNAP PEAS

THIS ASIAN-INSPIRED recipe is fast and delicious. More of a salad than a hot side, it contains just small amounts of the triggers sugar and scallions. It's a low-calorie, fresh and crunchy side for any plain entrée, and because it calls for frozen peas and snap peas, the fuss is nearly eliminated.

> 3 cups frozen peas, thawed
> 8 ounces frozen sugar snap peas, thawed
> ½ cup chopped scallions (as tolerated)
> 2 tablespoons sesame seeds
> 2 tablespoons light soy sauce
> 1 teaspoon sugar
> 2 tablespoons olive oil
> Salt to taste

1. Combine all ingredients in a medium bowl and toss well.
2. Serve immediately, or chill, covered, until ready to serve. Toss again just before serving.

MAKES 8 SERVINGS.

NUTRIENT ANALYSIS PER SERVING:

Calories (kcal) 106 ■ Protein (g) 4.4 ■ Carbohydrates (g) 11 ■ Fat (g) 4.8 ■ Saturated Fat (g) .6 ■ Sodium (mg) 217 ■ Cholesterol (mg) 0 ■ % Calories from Protein 18 ■ % Calories from Carbohydrates 45 ■ % Calories from Fat 43 ■ Total Dietary Fiber (g) 3.4

Herbed Oven Steak Fries

I'T'S HARD FOR anyone with GERD to rationalize eating French fries. They're deep fried, a no-no on any diet. Oven "frying" maintains the fresh potato taste, adds a little crispiness and, best of all, puts fries back on the menu. Many prefer the texture and taste of the potatoes unpeeled, but remove the peel if that's how you like them. Try making this same recipe with parsnips or sweet potatoes for variety. The herbs give the fries more flavor and eye appeal.

2 pounds Idaho or russet potatoes, well scrubbed
¼ cup vegetable oil
1 tablespoon dried parsley flakes
½ teaspoon dried oregano
½ teaspoon kosher salt
1 teaspoon paprika
½ teaspoon granulated garlic (as tolerated)
Nonstick olive oil cooking spray

1. Preheat oven to 425° F. Spray a baking sheet well with nonstick cooking spray. Set aside.
2. Cut the potatoes into ½-inch by 4-inch sticks and place in a large bowl (work quickly or the potatoes will brown).
3. Toss well with oil, parsley, oregano, salt, paprika, and garlic, if using.
4. Arrange the potatoes in a single layer on the prepared baking sheet. Spray the tops of the fries well with the olive oil spray.
5. Bake for 30–40 minutes, turning the potatoes once or twice, until golden and cooked through. Serve hot with added salt to taste.

MAKES 8 SERVINGS.

NUTRIENT ANALYSIS PER SERVING:

Calories (kcal) 129 ■ Protein (g) 2.3 ■ Carbohydrates (g) 14.5 ■ Fat (g) 7 ■ Saturated Fat (g) .7 ■ Sodium (mg) 99 ■ Cholesterol (mg) 0 ■ % Calories from Protein 7 ■ % Calories from Carbohydrates 45 ■ % Calories from Fat 49 ■ Total Dietary Fiber (g) 2

RISOTTO WITH SHIITAKE MUSHROOMS

RISOTTO, BASICALLY, IS rice, cooked slowly with small amounts of liquid added throughout the cooking process so that the finished dish has a creamy texture, without the cream, so there are few trigger foods involved. If you're uneasy about using onions or wine, leave the onions out and substitute more broth for the wine. The Parmesan cheese may be reduced or omitted as well, though, again, the amount is minimal. Technically, any rice may be made into risotto, but it's customary to use arborio, a short-grain Italian rice. There are countless recipes for risotto. This one includes shiitake mushrooms, though other mushrooms may be substituted.

1 cup dried shiitake mushrooms
5 cups fat-free, low-sodium chicken broth, boiling
2 tablespoons olive oil
½ cup chopped onions (as tolerated)
1 cup dry white wine
1 cup uncooked Italian arborio rice
Salt to taste
¼ cup fresh grated Parmesan cheese
¼ cup fresh minced parsley, garnish

1. Place mushrooms in a medium bowl. Pour 4 cups of the boiling broth over the mushrooms and allow them to stand for 20 minutes to soften (the remaining cup of broth need not be boiling). Remove the mushrooms from the broth with a slotted spoon and slice them into thin strips, discarding tough stems. Reserve the broth. Set aside.
2. Heat the oil in a medium nonstick skillet. Add the mushrooms and onions, if using. Sauté the mushrooms until lightly colored (and the onions are softened). Set aside.
3. Bring the broth used for soaking the mushrooms and wine to a boil in a medium saucepan over medium-high heat.
4. Add the arborio rice to the pan and bring to a boil.
5. Reduce heat immediately and simmer the rice, stirring occasionally, until most of the liquid is absorbed. Add the mushroom mixture. The rice must be creamy, but neither raw nor mushy. Continue cooking, adding additional broth if necessary to cook the rice through.

6. Add salt and cheese to the risotto and stir to melt the cheese. Serve the risotto hot, sprinkled with parsley.

MAKES 4–6 SERVINGS.

NUTRIENT ANALYSIS PER SERVING:

Calories (kcal) 410 ■ Protein (g) 16 ■ Carbohydrates (g) 55.5 ■ Fat (g) 10 ■ Saturated Fat (g) 2 ■ Sodium (mg) 428 ■ Cholesterol (mg) 35 ■ % Calories from Protein 16 ■ % Calories from Carbohydrates 54 ■ % Calories from Fat 23 ■ Total Dietary Fiber (g) 3

COCONUT RICE

Coconut milk is often left out of many fat-reduced recipes for good reason. Regular coconut milk is high in saturated fat and very caloric. Fortunately, lowfat and fat-free coconut milk is readily available in well-stocked markets and specialty stores. While coconut itself suffers from the same high-fat dilemma, the amount called for here is reduced from traditional coconut rice recipes.

> *1 cup unsweetened fat-free or lowfat coconut milk*
> *½ cup water*
> *¼ teaspoon salt*
> *1 cup long-grain white rice*
> *1 tablespoon white sesame seeds, lightly toasted*
> *¼ cup sweetened flaked coconut, lightly toasted*
> *¼ cup chopped scallions (as tolerated)*

1. Bring coconut milk, water, and salt to a boil in a small saucepan over medium-high heat.
2. Stir in the rice and bring the liquid to a boil again. Reduce heat and simmer the rice, covered, until the liquid is absorbed, about 15–20 minutes.
3. Stir in the sesame seeds. Transfer the rice to a serving bowl and sprinkle with toasted coconut and scallions, if using.

Makes 4 servings.

NUTRIENT ANALYSIS PER SERVING:

Calories (kcal) 247 ■ Protein (g) 4.7 ■ Carbohydrates (g) 43 ■ Fat (g) 6.4 ■ Saturated Fat (g) 4 ■ Sodium (mg) 179 ■ Cholesterol (mg) 0 ■ % Calories from Protein 8 ■ % Calories from Carbohydrates 70 ■ % Calories from Fat 24 ■ Total Dietary Fiber (g) 1.3

HORSERADISH MASHED YUKON GOLD POTATOES

Y UKON GOLD POTATOES with their golden yellow flesh are perfect mashing pota-toes. Fat-free sour cream makes the potatoes extra creamy without adding outrageous calories, so they work well if you're trying to keep your weight down. The small amount of horseradish will add just a touch of flavor to these already flavorful spuds. If you tolerate horseradish well, you may add more to your liking.

2 pounds Yukon gold potatoes, unpeeled, quartered
½ cup or more nonfat sour cream
1 tablespoon prepared white horseradish (as tolerated)
Salt to taste

1. Bring a large pot of water to a boil over high heat. Add potatoes and cook until very tender, about 25 minutes. Drain very well, but do not rinse.
2. Return potatoes to the hot empty pot. Using a masher or electric mixer, mash or beat the potatoes well.
3. Add remaining ingredients and mix well to incorporate. Adjust salt to taste and serve the potatoes hot or warm.

MAKES 6 SERVINGS.

--- NUTRIENT ANALYSIS PER SERVING: ---

Calories (kcal) 137 ■ Protein (g) 5.6 ■ Carbohydrates (g) 27 ■ Fat (g) 0.2 ■ Saturated Fat (g) 0 ■ Sodium (mg) 86 ■ Cholesterol (mg) 0 ■ % Calories from Protein 17 ■ % Calories from Carbohydrates 19 ■ % Calories from Fat 1 ■ Total Dietary Fiber (g) 2.3

Angel Hair Pasta with Blue Cheese, Honey, and Walnuts

THIS UNUSUAL PASTA is both savory and mildly sweet, and light, unlike creamy pastas that can contain dozens of fat grams and reflux-inducing garlic. Perfect as a foil for roast or grilled chicken or lean beef. The strong flavor of high-fat blue cheese means a little goes a long way, as in this recipe. Walnuts, though also high in fat, are used sparingly.

1 pound dry angel hair pasta or capellini
¼ cup olive oil
¼ cup honey
½ cup chopped walnuts, lightly toasted
1 cup crumbled Gorgonzola or Roquefort cheese
1 cup minced flat-leafed parsley leaves
Salt to taste

1. Bring a large pot of water to a boil over high heat.
2. Add the dry pasta to the boiling water and cook until al dente and, reserving two tablespoons of the cooking water, drain well.
3. In a small bowl, quickly combine the reserved water with the olive oil and honey and stir until smooth.
4. Toss the water and oil mixture with the pasta, walnuts, cheese, parsley, and salt to taste.

MAKES 8 SIDE DISH SERVINGS.

NUTRIENT ANALYSIS PER SERVING:

Calories (kcal) 413 ■ Protein (g) 12 ■ Carbohydrates (g) 53 ■ Fat (g) 17 ■ Saturated Fat (g) 4.6 ■ Sodium (mg) 262 ■ Cholesterol (mg) 12.7 ■ % Calories from Protein 12 ■ % Calories from Carbohydrates 52 ■ % Calories from Fat 37 ■ Total Dietary Fiber (g) 2

FRUITED NUTTED WILD RICE

WILD RICE IS really considered a grass, native to North America. Its nutty flavor is distinct and pairs easily with dried fruits and nuts. Many rice recipes call for cooking it in chicken broth and adding butter. Here water and olive oil are used instead, and apple cider boosts the flavor while keeping this chewy side dish vegetarian.

1 cup long-grain white rice
1 cup long-grain wild rice
8 cups water
¼ cup olive oil
½ cup apple cider or juice
½ cup pecans or walnuts, toasted and chopped
½ cup dried cherries or cranberries
1 cup chopped scallions, white and green parts (as tolerated)
Salt to taste
¼ cup fresh chopped parsley or 2 tablespoons dried parsley

1. Combine white rice and 2 cups of water in a saucepan over medium-high heat.
2. Bring the liquid to a boil, reduce heat to simmer, and cover the pan with a tight-fitting lid. Cook the rice until tender, about 20 minutes. Remove from heat and let cool.
3. Meanwhile, combine wild rice and 4 cups of water in a medium saucepan over medium-high heat.
4. Bring the liquid to a boil, reduce heat to simmer, and cover the pan with a tight-fitting lid. Cook the rice until tender, about 40 minutes, adding 1 to 2 cups of water if the original amount evaporates too quickly. Remove from heat, drain well if there is remaining liquid, and let cool (do not rinse the rice).
5. Combine both rices with the remaining ingredients in a large bowl and toss well. Adjust salt to taste and serve warm or at room temperature.

MAKES 12 SERVINGS.

_____ NUTRIENT ANALYSIS PER SERVING: _____

Calories (kcal) 202 ■ Protein (g) 3.7 ■ Carbohydrates (g) 30 ■ Fat (g) 7.8 ■ Saturated Fat (g) 1 ■ Sodium (mg) 52 ■ Cholesterol (mg) 0 ■ % Calories from Protein 7 ■ % Calories from Carbohydrates 59 ■ % Calories from Fat 35 ■ Total Dietary Fiber (g) 2

VEGETABLE KEBABS

Most vegetables are not GERD inducers. Tomatoes and onions are the most notorious exceptions. While some vegetables such as cabbage and broccoli may produce gas in the colon, they do not add to GERD. It's colorful and fun to arrange a variety of vegetables on skewers, but it's also great just to thread one type of vegetable on each skewer. Among the most popular vegetables for grilling are zucchini, bell peppers, mushrooms, carrots, and celery. If you decide to grill cherry tomatoes, note that they cook very quickly.

Vegetable chunks or pieces, sized and cut to your size preference
Olive oil to brush over veggies
Balsamic vinegar to drizzle over cooked veggies (as tolerated)
Kosher salt to taste
Dried or fresh chopped parsley to sprinkle over cooked kebabs

1. Preheat grill to medium-high.
2. Thread veggies (any variety) onto metal skewers or wooden or bamboo skewers (soak wooden or bamboo skewers in cold water for 1 hour or more first).
3. Brush the threaded vegetables with a little olive oil and grill, turning often, until the chunks are charred and cooked to your liking (hard vegetables, such as potatoes, may need to be cooked much longer, at a lower heat so they don't burn on the outside while remaining raw on the inside).
4. Serve the kebabs hot, warm, or at room temperature, drizzled with a little balsamic vinegar, salt, and sprinkled with parsley.

Makes as many servings as you wish.

For one kebab with 4 ounces of vegetables:

NUTRIENT ANALYSIS PER SERVING:

Calories (kcal) 58 ■ Protein (g) 1.2 ■ Carbohydrates (g) 8.7 ■ Fat (g) 2.4 ■ Saturated Fat (g) 0.3 ■ Sodium (mg) 83 ■ Cholesterol (mg) 0 ■ % Calories from Protein 8 ■ % Calories from Carbohydrates 60 ■ % Calories from Fat 38 ■ Total Dietary Fiber (g) 2.3

Roasted Eggplant and Red Peppers with Sesame Seeds

Even though eggplant is distantly related to the tomato, it doesn't possess tomato's reflux triggering properties. Roasting eggplant gives it an earthy, rich flavor. Though sometimes time-consuming to prepare, this recipe eliminates the need to salt and soak the eggplant before cooking. It's coupled with sweet bell pepper, which unlike its fiery cousin, the hot chili pepper, is safe to eat in moderation.

Olive oil for brushing eggplant slices
1 large (1½–2 pounds) eggplant, unpeeled, cut crosswise into ½-inch-thick rounds
2 red bell peppers, sliced into thin strips, lengthwise
Fine sea salt to taste
1 teaspoon sesame oil
¼ teaspoon dried oregano
2 tablespoons sesame seeds
Juice of ½ lemon (as tolerated)
½ cup fresh minced parsley
½ cup Niçoise or Kalamata black olives

1. Preheat oven to 500°. Brush baking sheet very lightly with olive oil.
2. Arrange eggplant slices in a single layer on the baking sheet and brush the tops with olive oil. Roast for 10 minutes, turning once after 5 minutes.
3. Arrange red pepper strips over the eggplant and sprinkle with salt. Drizzle sesame oil and sprinkle oregano over the peppers. Roast for 5 minutes more.
4. Sprinkle sesame seeds over and roast for 2 minutes more.
5. Remove from oven and let the vegetables cool before transferring them to a serving dish. Drizzle the lemon juice, if using, and sprinkle with minced parsley. Garnish with olives and serve as a first course or side dish with pita wedges.

Makes 6–8 servings.

NUTRIENT ANALYSIS PER SERVING:

Calories (kcal) 135 ■ Protein (g) 2 ■ Carbohydrates (g) 10.6 ■ Fat (g) 10.4 ■ Saturated Fat (g) 1.4 ■ Sodium (mg) 128 ■ Cholesterol (mg) 0 ■ % Calories from Protein 6 ■ % Calories from Carbohydrates 32 ■ % Calories from Fat 70 ■ Total Dietary Fiber (g) 4.1

Asparagus with Tahini Yogurt Dressing

Asparagus is most often eaten plain—steamed with just a bit of butter. This recipe adds a light sauce with the Middle Eastern flavor of tahini, a thick spread made from ground sesame seeds. Though it's high in fat, it's used in small amounts as a condiment, adding the nutty, satisfying flavor of sesame. For variety, quickly blanch the asparagus and use double the amount of dressing as a dipping sauce.

> *2 pounds asparagus, trimmed*
> *Water*

DRESSING:
> *1 cup nonfat plain yogurt or tofu yogurt*
> *3 tablespoons tahini (sesame paste)*
> *1 tablespoon olive oil*
> *½ teaspoon kosher salt*

1. Cook asparagus: Bring a pan of salted water to a boil over high heat. Add trimmed asparagus and cook until tender, but still very green, about 3–5 minutes.
2. Drain asparagus quickly and rinse with cold water to stop the cooking process. Drain well again and dry with paper towels before arranging on a serving plate.
3. Make dressing: Combine all ingredients in a small bowl and whisk until smooth. Chill until ready to serve.
4. Drizzle the dressing, to taste, over the asparagus spears just before serving.

MAKES 8 SERVINGS.

NUTRIENT ANALYSIS PER SERVING:

Calories (kcal) 89 ■ Protein (g) 5.2 ■ Carbohydrates (g) 3.9 ■ Fat (g) 5.7 ■ Saturated Fat (g) 0 ■ Sodium (mg) 129 ■ Cholesterol (mg) 0.5 ■ % Calories from Protein 24 ■ % Calories from Carbohydrates 18 ■ % Calories from Fat 58 ■ Total Dietary Fiber (g) 1

Basmati Rice with Peas and Pistachios

Basmati rice is used most often in Asian cooking. A long-grain rice, it has a nutty, almost sweet flavor of its own. Paired with stomach-calming fresh gingerroot and high-fiber peas and pistachios, this rice could really be a meal in itself.

2 cups uncooked brown basmati rice, rinsed well and drained
5 cups water
3 tablespoons olive oil
2 tablespoons minced fresh gingerroot
2 teaspoons dry mustard (as tolerated)
1 teaspoon turmeric
Salt to taste
2 cups fresh or frozen peas, thawed
½ cup, or more, shelled pistachios, toasted to taste

1. Combine rice and water in a medium saucepan over medium-high heat. Bring the water to a boil, reduce the heat, and cover the pan. Cook 30–40 minutes until the water is absorbed and the rice is tender. Remove the pan from the heat and set aside.
2. While the rice is cooking, heat oil in large nonstick skillet over medium-high heat. Add the gingerroot, mustard, turmeric, salt, and peas, stirring frequently for 3 minutes more.
3. Add the skillet mixture to the pan of cooked rice and stir to combine and coat the rice with the mixture.
4. Carefully fold in half of the nuts and stir again. Serve the rice garnished with the remaining nuts.

Makes 8 servings.

Nutrient Analysis Per Serving:

Calories (kcal) 287 ▪ Protein (g) 7.5 ▪ Carbohydrates (g) 42 ▪ Fat (g) 10 ▪ Saturated Fat (g) 1.5 ▪ Sodium (mg) 137 ▪ Cholesterol (mg) 0 ▪ % Calories from Protein 10 ▪ % Calories from Carbohydrates 59 ▪ % Calories from Fat 32 ▪ Total Dietary Fiber (g) 4.2

CURRIED STUFFED NEW POTATOES

Small new potatoes are halved and hollowed into little cups to hold a flavorful mixture of potatoes, raisins, and nuts. The filling is seasoned with curry, a blend of many spices, which, depending on the manufacturer, can be quite spicy hot. Look for mild curry to use in this recipe. Used in small amounts, as in this recipe, you'll get the flavor of the spice mix, without the discomfort that can be associated with many foods containing higher amounts of especially hot curry. Gingerroot, soothing to GERD sufferers, also adds exotic flavor to this dish.

12 small new potatoes, boiled and cut in half
3 tablespoons olive oil
2 teaspoons minced fresh gingerroot
1–2 teaspoons curry powder (as tolerated)
¼ cup golden raisins
2 tablespoons chopped pecans
2 tablespoons apple juice or cider
Kosher salt to taste

1. Preheat oven to 350° F. Spray a baking sheet with nonstick cooking spray. Cut cooked potatoes in half and scoop out insides (leave enough of the flesh to keep the potato skin intact.)
2. Heat oil in a large nonstick skillet over medium-high heat. Add potato flesh and remaining ingredients and heat through, using a fork or spoon to break up the potato into smaller pieces.
3. Spoon the hot potato mixture back into the potato shells and place on the prepared baking sheet.
4. Bake the potatoes, uncovered, for 10–15 minutes until hot.

Makes 24 potato halves.

NUTRIENT ANALYSIS PER SERVING:

Calories (kcal) 50 ■ Protein (g) 1 ■ Carbohydrates (g) 7 ■ Fat (g) 2 ■ Saturated Fat (g) 0 ■ Sodium (mg) 13 ■ Cholesterol (mg) 0 ■ % Calories from Protein 8 ■ % Calories from Carbohydrates 55 ■ % Calories from Fat 38 ■ Total Dietary Fiber (g) .8

Roasted Yams with Rosemary and Balsamic Vinegar

DON'T BE AFRAID of the vinegar in the name of this recipe. There's just enough to add flavor, and since it's distributed among the four pounds of potatoes, fairly harmless to most GERD sufferers. The same holds true for the herbs used here. While this recipe calls for rosemary, tarragon, and sage, substitute your favorite herbs for variety.

4 pounds yams or sweet potatoes, peeled and cut into 1-inch chunks
⅓ cup olive oil
1 tablespoon dried rosemary, or to taste
2 teaspoons dried tarragon
1 teaspoon dried crumbled sage
1 teaspoon kosher salt, or to taste
2 tablespoons balsamic vinegar (as tolerated)

1. Preheat oven to 425° F. Combine all ingredients except balsamic vinegar in large bowl. Toss well to coat the yams.
2. Transfer the yams to a large baking dish. Roast the vegetables, uncovered, until tender, about 1 hour, turning them once or twice.
3. Drizzle the yams with the balsamic and roast for 10 minutes more. Adjust salt to taste and serve hot.

MAKES 12 SERVINGS.

NUTRIENT ANALYSIS PER SERVING:

Calories (kcal) 179 ▪ Protein (g) 2 ▪ Carbohydrates (g) 30 ▪ Fat (g) 6 ▪ Saturated Fat (g) 1 ▪ Sodium (mg) 158 ▪ Cholesterol (mg) 0 ▪ % Calories from Protein 5 ▪ % Calories from Carbohydrates 66 ▪ % Calories from Fat 31 ▪ Total Dietary Fiber (g) 3.7

ISRAELI COUSCOUS WITH ROASTED RED PEPPERS AND CHICKPEAS

ISRAELI COUSCOUS IS different—much larger in size, like small round pellets or beads, and lightly toasted—than the tiny Northern African couscous you may be used to. Look for it in Middle Eastern markets or well-stocked supermarkets. You can also make this recipe with the smaller couscous, cutting the amount of liquid by one cup and cooking the couscous for about 3 minutes instead of 8. This recipe calls for celery or fresh tomatoes, if you can tolerate them. The bell pepper, unlike hot peppers, doesn't have the same effect of GERD sufferers.

> 1 red bell pepper, roasted (see below), or jarred roasted red pepper
> 3 tablespoons olive oil
> ½ cup diced celery or tomatoes
> 2 cups Israeli couscous
> 4 cups boiling water or fat-free, low-sodium chicken broth
> 1 cup cooked chickpeas
> 2 tablespoons dried parsley flakes or ½ cup fresh minced parsley
> Kosher salt to taste

1. Roast pepper:
   Gas stove roasting of peppers: Cut the bell pepper in half, lengthwise and remove white membrane and seeds. If you have a gas stove, turn the heat to high and turn on the overhead fan. Place the pepper, skin side down over the flame and char the skin until blackened—you will have to move the peppers around to char them completely. Cool slightly and rub off most of the charred skin. (It helps to place the peppers in a foil packet to cool—this loosens the skin even more.)
   Oven roasting of peppers: Preheat oven to broil and move rack to just above center. Place pepper, cut side down, on a baking sheet. Broil until the skin is very blackened, about 10–12 minutes. Cool slightly and rub off most of the charred skin. (It helps to place the peppers in a foil packet to cool—this loosens the skin even more.)
2. Dice the roasted pepper and set aside.
3. Meanwhile, heat oil in a large saucepan over medium-high heat. Add the celery or tomatoes and couscous and cook for 3–4 minutes more, stirring frequently, until the couscous is lightly colored.
4. Add the boiling water, chickpeas, and parsley and stir well. Cover and cook the couscous for 8–12 minutes, until the water is absorbed.

5. Stir in the red bell pepper, season to taste with salt, and serve hot as a side dish.

Makes 8 servings.

Nutrient Analysis Per Serving:

Calories (kcal) 231 ▪ Protein (g) 6.6 ▪ Carbohydrates (g) 37 ▪ Fat (g) 5.9 ▪ Saturated Fat (g) .7 ▪ Sodium (mg) 82 ▪ Cholesterol (mg) 0 ▪ % Calories from Protein 11 ▪ % Calories from Carbohydrates 65 ▪ % Calories from Fat 23 ▪ Total Dietary Fiber (g) 3.8

CANDIED CARROTS

CARROTS ARE EXTREMELY high in fiber—a perfect food for GERD sufferers. Unlike many recipes for calorie-rich, buttery, sticky-sweet candied or glazed carrots, this one makes lightly glazed carrots for optimum flavor and reduced calories and fat.

> *2 tablespoons olive oil*
> *1 pound peeled baby carrots, sliced once diagonally*
> *1 tablespoon brown sugar*
> *2 tablespoons honey*
> *1 tablespoon dried parsley flakes*
> *Kosher salt to taste*

1. Heat oil in a large nonstick skillet over medium-high heat.
2. Add carrots and sauté for 3 minutes. Add the brown sugar and honey and cook, stirring frequently, until the sugar dissolves.
3. Stir in the parsley, reduce heat, and cook the carrots, carefully stirring frequently, until the carrots are tender and glazed. Season with a little salt and serve hot.

MAKES 4 SERVINGS.

NUTRIENT ANALYSIS PER SERVING:

Calories (kcal) 148 ■ Protein (g) 1 ■ Carbohydrates (g) 21 ■ Fat (g) 7.3 ■ Saturated Fat (g) 1 ■ Sodium (mg) 68 ■ Cholesterol (mg) 0 ■ % Calories from Protein 3 ■ % Calories from Carbohydrates 58 ■ % Calories from Fat 45 ■ Total Dietary Fiber (g) 2

LAYERED MAPLE SWEET POTATOES WITH PECANS

SWEET POTATOES NEED very little added to make them delicious. This recipe creates a candied version of this favorite spud. What's different is that fat has been reduced to a minimum, and soothing gingerroot had been added for a flavor boost.

2½–3 pounds sweet potatoes (all potatoes similar in size)
2 tablespoons butter
¼ cup brown sugar
¼ cup real maple syrup
1 tablespoon minced gingerroot
½ teaspoon salt
1 tablespoon fresh minced sage or ½ teaspoon dried sage
¼ cup flour
¼ cup chopped pecans, lightly toasted

1. Preheat oven to 375° F. Spray a 9-inch glass or ceramic pie plate with nonstick cooking spray.
2. Peel the sweet potatoes and cut them into thin slices (about ¼-inch). Transfer the sliced potatoes into a large bowl. Set aside.
3. Combine butter, brown sugar, maple syrup, gingerroot, salt, sage, and flour in a small saucepan over medium heat. Cook, stirring frequently until the sugar dissolves, about 3 minutes. Pour this over the potatoes and toss to coat the potatoes well.
4. Arrange sweet potatoes in circles around the pie dish, overlapping the slices as necessary. Cover the dish with foil.
5. Bake the potatoes for 1 hour. Remove foil and bake for 30 minutes more.
6. Remove from oven, sprinkle with pecans, cut into wedges, and serve.

MAKES 8 SERVINGS.

NUTRIENT ANALYSIS PER SERVING:

Calories (kcal) 242 ■ Protein (g) 3 ■ Carbohydrates (g) 46.7 ■ Fat (g) 5.5 ■ Saturated Fat (g) 2 ■ Sodium (mg) 193 ■ Cholesterol (mg) 8.2 ■ % Calories from Protein 5 ■ % Calories from Carbohydrates 77 ■ % Calories from Fat 21 ■ Total Dietary Fiber (g) 4

Main Event

EVERYDAY EATING HAS two requirements. First, the food must be accessible, or easily purchased near your home. Next, they must be able to be made quickly and easily.

Most of the entrées here include regular grocery items. While some may include a few gourmet or ethnic ingredients, these items are becoming increasingly available—if not, you can substitute other ingredients. Button mushrooms or shiitake mushrooms can be used instead of morel mushrooms, for instance.

We've made preparation simple, even with some recipes requiring many ingredients, because we know that recipes requiring too much fussing won't be made often. For many of the dishes here, the longest part of the preparation time is waiting for them to cook.

We also recommend investing in a good set of nonstick cookware. While it's not the professional chef's choice for cooking, for those with GERD, nonstick translates into less fat needed for cooking—perfect for those trying to lose weight and for those avoiding fatty foods, known reflux triggers.

We've included recipes for dressier, elegant entrées. There are recipes for trendier dishes, the kind you'll find at stylish, newer restaurants. You'll also find comforting, traditional recipes for many family favorites, made over to be safe for GERD sufferers. We've pointed out how each recipe differs in preparation from the "regular" way—a way that could cause distress. All in all, we've eliminated many trigger foods and lightened calorie and fat counts considerably.

Among the most important thing to remember when eating any entrée—or any food for that matter—is that portion size counts. Eating too much, even of the most harmless foods, can cause reflux. As stated earlier in the book, large quantities can weaken the LES, allowing GERD to ensue.

Read on for recipes for seafood, beef, chicken, pork, lamb, pasta, and vegetarian entrée dishes.

SEARED SCALLOPS
WITH CARROTS, ZUCCHINI, AND PARSLEY

Sea scallops are light and meaty—low in both calories and cholesterol. Scallops are often available breaded and deep fried, a bad choice for GERD sufferers. We've taken away the breading and used zucchini instead of the tomatoes normally called for in this recipe, and reduced the amounts of garlic and wine, so it's safer to eat. While some enjoy scallops rare, and others cooked to a crisp, they're best served at medium, seared with a crisp, brown crust.

> 4 tablespoons olive oil
> 1/2 teaspoon fresh minced garlic (as tolerated)
> 1 cup 1/4-inch diced carrots
> 1 1/2 cups diced, unpeeled zucchini
> 1/2 cup fresh minced parsley
> 2 tablespoons light soy sauce
> 1/4 cup dry white wine
> 20 large fresh sea scallops (about 1-inch thickness)
> Kosher salt to taste

1. Heat 2 tablespoons of the oil in a large nonstick skillet over high heat.
2. Add the garlic, if using, and carrots. Cook, stirring constantly, until the carrots begin to color, about 3 minutes.
3. Add the zucchini and parsley and cook for 2 minutes more. Add the soy sauce and wine and cook for 2 minutes more. Season to taste with salt and set aside.
4. Dry scallops with paper towel to remove excess moisture.
5. Heat remaining 2 tablespoons of the oil until hot in a large nonstick skillet over high heat.
6. Add the scallops and sear them for about 2 minutes on each side for medium-rare.
7. Arrange the scallops on 4 dinner-sized plates and spoon the warm carrot and zucchini sauce over. Sprinkle with more salt if desired and serve immediately.

MAKES 4 SERVINGS.

NUTRIENT ANALYSIS PER SERVING:

Calories (kcal) 229 ■ Protein (g) 12.4 ■ Carbohydrates (g) 8 ■ Fat (g) 16 ■ Saturated Fat (g) 1.8 ■ Sodium (mg) 602 ■ Cholesterol (mg) 20.7 ■ % Calories from Protein 22 ■ % Calories from Carbohydrates 13 ■ % Calories from Fat 62 ■ Total Dietary Fiber (g) 1.7

Foil-Baked Sea Bass
with Morel Mushroom Sauce

Sᴇᴀ ʙᴀꜱꜱ ɪꜱ the current seafood culinary darling. After all, it is mild, hearty, flavorful, and infinitely adaptable. Like most fish, sea bass is a lowfat source of heart-healthy, omega-3 fats. This recipe removes much of the fat and calories in traditional mushroom cream sauces. If you choose not to use wine in the recipe, substitute fat-free chicken or vegetable broth instead.

Mᴜꜱʜʀᴏᴏᴍ Sᴀᴜᴄᴇ:
> 6–10 dried morels or fresh morel mushrooms
> Hot water
> 1 cup dry white wine (as tolerated)
> ¼ cup finely chopped shallots (as tolerated)
> ½ cup fat-free half-and-half
> ½ cup fat-free chicken or vegetable broth
> ½ teaspoon dried thyme or 2 teaspoons fresh thyme
> 8 ounces button mushrooms, sliced
> Kosher salt to taste

Fɪꜱʜ:
> 4 6- to 8-ounce sea bass fillets (each about 1½ inches thick)
> 2 tablespoons extra virgin olive oil
> Kosher salt to taste
> ½ cup fresh chopped basil or parsley

1. Make sauce: If using dried mushrooms, soak dried morels in one cup of hot (not boiling) water for 30 minutes. Drain well and slice into rings. Set aside. If using fresh mushrooms, slice into rings and set aside.
2. Simmer wine and shallots, if using, in a large nonstick skillet over medium heat until liquid is reduced to about two tablespoons.
3. Add half-and-half and simmer for another minute.
4. Add morels, button mushrooms, broth, and thyme, then simmer for 5 minutes. Keep the sauce warm until ready to serve.
5. Assemble the fish: Preheat oven to 475°F. Cut four sheets of foil, each about 14 inches long. Lay one sheet of foil, shiny side down, on a flat surface. Place one piece of fish on one half of the foil.

6. Drizzle the fish with a little of the olive oil and season with salt. Top with a fourth of the fresh basil or parsley. Fold other half of foil over the fish and seal the edges well to form a packet.
7. Place the packet on a baking sheet. Repeat with remaining fish. Bake fish until just cooked through, about 15 minutes.
8. Place fish packets on plates. Open the packets by carefully unfolding the foil and spoon the warm mushroom sauce over (you may serve in the open foil packets or remove the fish to dinner plates).

MAKES 4 SERVINGS.

NUTRIENT ANALYSIS PER SERVING:

Calories (kcal) 308 ■ Protein (g) 41 ■ Carbohydrates (g) 6.4 ■ Fat (g) 12.7 ■ Saturated Fat (g) 2.2 ■ Sodium (mg) 252 ■ Cholesterol (mg) 82.5 ■ % Calories from Protein 53 ■ % Calories from Carbohydrates 8 ■ % Calories from Fat 37 ■ Total Dietary Fiber (g) 1

Poached Salmon Fillets with Mediterranean Vegetables

Most salmon we buy in this country is farm-raised with tremendous eye-appeal due to its bright pinkish color. And like most other fish, it's low in calories and high in omega-3s for heart health. We've made this GERD-safe salmon by reducing the amounts of wine, tomatoes, and vinegar, and substituting zucchini and white beans for more fiber, with or without the vegetables. Serve it simply with a sauce of fat-free yogurt (as tolerated), diced cucumber, fresh chopped dill, and a little salt. The vegetables are also wonderful as a side salad or tossed with fresh hot or cold pasta.

> 4 (5- or 6 ounce) salmon fillets (1-inch thick)
> Water
> ½ cup dry white wine (as tolerated)
> ½ cup diced plum tomatoes (as tolerated)
> 2 cups diced, unpeeled zucchini
> 1 cup finely chopped seeded peeled cucumber
> 1 cup cooked white beans or great northern beans, drained (canned is fine)
> ¼ cup coarsely chopped Kalamata olives
> ¼ cup chopped scallions (as tolerated)
> 1 tablespoon drained capers
> 2 tablespoons balsamic vinegar (as tolerated)
> Kosher salt to taste
> 12 fresh basil leaves

1. Fill a large nonstick skillet or pot with 2 inches of water and ½ cup wine, if using.
2. Bring to a boil over high heat.
3. Add salmon fillets and bring the liquid to a boil again. Reduce heat immediately and cover pot. Cook the salmon for 7 minutes. Remove from heat and leave the salmon in the pan to cool slightly.
4. Carefully transfer the salmon to a shallow dish, cover with plastic wrap, and chill up to one day.
5. Combine tomatoes (if using), zucchini, cucumbers, beans, olives, scallions (if using), and capers in a large bowl. Toss well to combine. Add the vinegar and salt to taste.

6. To serve, arrange cold salmon fillets on 4 individual dinner-sized plates. Spoon ¼ of the tomato mixture around each of the salmon fillets. Garnish the fish with the basil leaves.

MAKES 4 SERVINGS.

──────── NUTRIENT ANALYSIS PER SERVING: ────────

Calories (kcal) 346 ■ Protein (g) 36 ■ Carbohydrates (g) 16 ■ Fat (g) 14 ■ Saturated Fat (g) 2.4 ■ Sodium (mg) 416 ■ Cholesterol (mg) 102 ■ % Calories from Protein 42 ■ % Calories from Carbohydrates 18 ■ % Calories from Fat 37 ■ Total Dietary Fiber (g) 4.6

GRILLED MUSTARD-BASTED SHRIMP KEBABS

M USTARD MAY BE an irritant to some people with GERD, so if you can't tolerate it, leave it out of this recipe. Many are able to enjoy small amounts, as in this savory, luxurious shrimp dish. Other GERD inducers such as onions, garlic, and lemon juice have been eliminated from this recipe, and fresh gingerroot, safe for those with reflux, replaces the flavor lost. You may also skip the skewers and simply broil or sear these shrimp if you wish.

BASTING SAUCE:

>   2 tablespoons minced fresh gingerroot
>   1 tablespoon brown sugar
>   1 tablespoon Dijon mustard (as tolerated)
>   3 tablespoons olive oil
>   1 tablespoon Worcestershire sauce
>   1 tablespoon dried parsley flakes

>   40 very large (25–30 per pound) raw shrimp, peeled, and deveined,
>   tail left on
>   8 long metal skewers or 8 bamboo skewers (10-inches long or more),
>   soaked an hour or more in water

1. Prepare basting sauce: Whisk together the basting sauce ingredients and set aside.
2. Heat grill to medium-high.
3. Thread 5 shrimp per skewer (you may wish to use two skewers per kebab so that the shrimp don't spin on the skewers).
4. Baste one side of kebabs with basting sauce and grill the kebabs, basted side down, until lightly cooked, about 3 minutes.
5. Brush unbasted side of the kebabs with basting sauce and turn to grill other side. Grill kebabs until underside is lightly charred, about 3 minutes more. Discard unused basting sauce.
6. Immediately serve the kebabs if you want to eat them hot, or serve at room temperature.

M AKES 8 SERVINGS.

NUTRIENT ANALYSIS PER SERVING:

Calories (kcal) 112.5 ■ Protein (g) 12 ■ Carbohydrates (g) 2.5 ■ Fat (g) 5.8 ■ Saturated Fat (g) .86 ■ Sodium (mg) 160 ■ Cholesterol (mg) 110.6 ■ % Calories from Protein 43 ■ % Calories from Carbohydrates 9 ■ % Calories from Fat 47 ■ Total Dietary Fiber (g) 0

Seared Tuna with Raisins and Capers

Aɴ ᴜɴᴜsᴜᴀʟ ᴄᴏᴍʙɪɴᴀᴛɪᴏɴ that features two favorite tastes—sweet and savory. For variety, use any type of steak fish: salmon and swordfish work well. For variation, you could also add toasted pine nuts or almonds for more fiber. GERD-inciter wine has been reduced considerably and can be replaced by chicken broth if desired. The mildly sweet and sour flavors of the raisins replace the savory tastes of garlic and onions here.

¼ cup golden raisins
½ cup boiling water
4 tuna steaks (6 to 7 ounces each)
½ cup flour
¼ cup olive oil
½ cup dry white wine
½ cup chopped celery
½ cup fresh chopped parsley, divided
1 tablespoon drained capers
1 bay leaf, crumbled
¼ teaspoon ground cinnamon (as tolerated)
Kosher salt

1. Place raisins in small bowl and cover with boiling water. Soak the raisins for 30 minutes and drain. Set aside.
2. Dredge tuna in flour and pat lightly with your hands to remove excess flour.
3. Heat olive oil until very hot in a large nonstick skillet over high heat.
4. Add the tuna, and brown it well on both sides.
5. Carefully pour the wine into the pan, add the celery, half the parsley, capers, bay leaf, cinnamon, and soaked raisins (discard water). Bring the liquid to a boil and cook until it is reduced by half, about 3 minutes.
6. Serve the tuna immediately, with sauce spooned over and sprinkled with kosher salt and remaining parsley.

Mᴀᴋᴇs 4 sᴇʀᴠɪɴɢs.

Nᴜᴛʀɪᴇɴᴛ Aɴᴀʟʏsɪs Pᴇʀ Sᴇʀᴠɪɴɢ:

Calories (kcal) 433 ■ Protein (g) 36 ■ Carbohydrates (g) 21 ■ Fat (g) 20.8 ■ Saturated Fat (g) 3.7 ■ Sodium (mg) 191 ■ Cholesterol (mg) 55.5 ■ % Calories from Protein 33 ■ % Calories from Carbohydrates 19 ■ % Calories from Fat 43 ■ Total Dietary Fiber (g) 1.7

ROAST SALMON WITH FENNEL AND WHITE WINE

I F YOU LOVE fennel, you'll love this recipe. Roasting this large, celery-like vegetable gives it an earthy flavor. And when you slice fennel thin, as in this recipe, it resembles sliced onions, which have been excluded from this dish. Wine, garlic, and mustard have been greatly reduced to safer amounts, but feel free to reduce these ingredients further or substitute chicken or vegetable broth for the wine in this recipe.

SALMON:

2½ to 3 pounds salmon fillet, bones removed
   (may also be cut into 6 portions)
1 large fennel bulb, halved vertically and sliced very thin
2 tablespoons olive oil, plus 1 additional tablespoon oil
1 tablespoon Dijon mustard (as tolerated)
½ teaspoon minced garlic (as tolerated)
1½ cups bread crumbs
½ cup fresh chopped parsley
1 cup dry white wine
Kosher salt

1. Prepare fish: Preheat oven to 400°F. Spray a baking sheet with sides with non-stick cooking spray.
2. Arrange the salmon fillet (or pieces of fish) on the baking sheet. Separate the fennel into slices and arrange around the fish.
3. Combine 2 tablespoons of the oil, mustard, and garlic, if using, in a small bowl and whisk well. Brush the oil and mustard mixture over the fish and season with a little salt.
4. Sprinkle the breadcrumbs and parsley over the fish and pour the white wine around the fillet.
5. Drizzle the remaining tablespoon of oil over the fennel. Season well with kosher salt. Do not cover with foil.
6. Place the baking sheet in the preheated oven and cook for 10 minutes (a couple of minutes longer if the fish is very thick).
7. Remove the fish from the oven and, using a baking sheet with no sides as a large spatula, remove the whole fillet to a serving platter. Arrange fennel around the

fish. (Or remove the fish pieces to a platter or individual serving plates and arrange fennel around.) Serve immediately.

MAKES 6 SERVINGS.

NUTRIENT ANALYSIS PER SERVING:

Calories (kcal) 528 ■ Protein (g) 47 ■ Carbohydrates (g) 23.4 ■ Fat (g) 25.6 ■ Saturated Fat (g) 4.2 ■ Sodium (mg) 420 ■ Cholesterol (mg) 135.6 ■ % Calories from Protein 35 ■ % Calories from Carbohydrates 18 ■ % Calories from Fat 44 ■ Total Dietary Fiber (g) 2

SEVEN VEGETABLE MOROCCAN-STYLE COUSCOUS

COUSCOUS IS THE national dish of Morocco and a wonderful tiny pasta that cooks in minutes in hot liquid. A good alternative to rice or potatoes, this recipe is low in calories, with fiber from the vegetables and beans. Leeks and fresh tomatoes, though reduced in amounts, can be eliminated, if they trigger episodes of GERD. Cilantro has a calming effect on acids, but if it's not a flavor you prefer, substitute fresh parsley instead. This couscous can be made vegetarian by substituting chicken-flavored bouillon or vegetable broth in place of the chicken broth.

¼ cup plus 1 tablespoon olive oil
2 large leeks (white and pale green parts only) sliced thin
   (as tolerated)
5 cups fat-free, low-sodium chicken broth
1 cup peeled butternut squash cut into ½-inch cubes,
   or sweet potatoes
1 large yellow squash, cut into ½-inch cubes
1 large zucchini cut into ½-inch cubes
¾ cup frozen baby lima beans, thawed
1 teaspoon turmeric
½ teaspoon ground ginger
Kosher salt to taste
1 cup diced seeded plum tomatoes (as tolerated)
¾ cup frozen peas, thawed
½ cup coarsely chopped fresh cilantro
1½ cups (about 10 ounces) dry couscous
½ cup slivered almonds, lightly toasted, garnish
1½ cup golden raisins, garnish

1. Heat ¼ cup oil in heavy large pan or Dutch oven over low heat. Add the leeks. Cover the pot and cook until the leeks are very tender but not brown, stirring occasionally, for about 10 minutes.
2. Add 2 cups of the chicken broth, butternut squash, yellow squash, zucchini, lima beans, turmeric, and ginger and stir to combine. Season the vegetables with salt to taste.
3. Increase the heat to medium-high and bring the mixture to boil.

4. Cover, reduce heat to medium and simmer until vegetables are crisp-tender, about 5 minutes.
5. Stir in tomatoes (if using), peas, and cilantro. Reduce heat to its lowest setting to keep warm while you make the couscous.
6. Make the couscous: In a large saucepan with a tight-fitting lid, bring remaining 3 cups of broth to a boil over high heat. Add couscous, stir, and cover. Remove from heat and let stand 10 minutes.
7. Fluff couscous with a fork before transferring it to a large platter. Arrange vegetable mixture over the couscous and garnish with the almonds and golden raisins.

MAKES 8 SERVINGS.

NUTRIENT ANALYSIS PER SERVING:

Calories (kcal) 381 ■ Protein (g) 14 ■ Carbohydrates (g) 50 ■ Fat (g) 14.4 ■ Saturated Fat (g) 1.7 ■ Sodium (mg) 212 ■ Cholesterol (mg) 15.6 ■ % Calories from Protein 15 ■ % Calories from Carbohydrates 52 ■ % Calories from Fat 34 ■ Total Dietary Fiber (g) 7

SLOW-COOKED LAMB CHOPS WITH OREGANO

LAMB AND OREGANO are great partners in this tender stew-like entrée. This recipe is easily customized by varying the herbs or adding extra ingredients such as diced carrots, celery, or potatoes. While the meal is flavorful, it is not very spicy, as many lamb dishes tend to be. That's because we've eliminated garlic and fresh lemon juice, which are often paired with lamb. You can replace the wine with extra broth if you wish.

8 large lamb chops or steaks with bones
1 teaspoon kosher salt
½ cup apple cider or juice
Grated peel or zest from 1 lemon (as tolerated)
2 teaspoons dried oregano
3 tablespoons extra virgin olive oil
3 bay leaves
1 cup white wine (as tolerated)
1 cup chicken broth
Fresh chopped parsley, garnish

1. Place lamb in a glass baking dish and season it to taste with salt.
2. Drizzle apple cider over the lamb and sprinkle the grated peel, if using, and oregano over. Drizzle the olive oil over all and place the bay leaves between a couple of the chops.
3. Cover the dish with plastic wrap and refrigerate for 4 hours or more.
4. Preheat oven to 325°F.
5. Heat a nonstick skillet over high heat. Remove the lamb from the marinade and brown on both sides before placing the chops back into the baking dish with the marinade.
6. Pour in the wine and broth. Cover the dish with foil and cook for 2 or more hours until the meat is very tender. Garnish with parsley and serve hot.

MAKES 6 SERVINGS.

--- NUTRIENT ANALYSIS PER SERVING: ---

Calories (kcal) 434 ■ Protein (g) 49 ■ Carbohydrates (g) 1.6 ■ Fat (g) 24 ■ Saturated Fat (g) 7 ■ Sodium (mg) 487 ■ Cholesterol (mg) 165 ■ % Calories from Protein 45 ■ % Calories from Carbohydrates 2 ■ % Calories from Fat 49 ■ Total Dietary Fiber (g) .3

GRILLED MARINATED FLANK STEAK

Flank steak, cooked medium rare, is such a treat. This recipe is easy to prepare and satisfying, especially when served with horseradish mashed potatoes (page 171). And because it's grilled quickly, you aren't spending hours fussing over a stove. Since flank steak is not an expensive cut of beef, it's affordable enough to make for a crowd. Though this recipe contains a minimal amount of garlic, you may still wish to cook without it. Soothing gingerroot and cilantro may also offset the effects of garlic.

> *3–4 pounds flank steak*
> *¼ cup olive oil*
> *½ cup light soy sauce*
> *2 tablespoons brown sugar*
> *½ teaspoon fresh minced garlic (as tolerated)*
> *2 tablespoons fresh minced gingerroot*
> *1 cup chopped red bell pepper*
> *½ cup fresh chopped cilantro*

1. Place uncut flank steak into a large dish or plastic zipper bag to marinate.
2. Combine remaining ingredients in a medium bowl and whisk well. Pour this mixture over the meat and turn the meat until it is well coated. Marinate meat, turning occasionally 2 hours or up to overnight.
3. Heat grill to medium-high. Remove the meat from the marinade and grill for 5 minutes on each side for medium-rare (discard marinade), or longer for less rare beef.
4. Let stand a minute or two before cutting the steak into ¼-inch slices against the grain.

MAKES 8 SERVINGS.

NUTRIENT ANALYSIS PER SERVING:

Calories (kcal) 475 ■ Protein (g) 52 ■ Carbohydrates (g) 2.7 ■ Fat (g) 27 ■ Saturated Fat (g) 10.7 ■ Sodium (mg) 362 ■ Cholesterol (mg) 132 ■ % Calories from Protein 44 ■ % Calories from Carbohydrates 2 ■ % Calories from Fat 51 ■ Total Dietary Fiber (g) 0

Turkey "Meatloaf"

Meatloaf is one of those foods that's normally not very healthful, often made with high fat-content meat and whole eggs. It also customarily includes large amounts of onions, garlic, and tomato paste or sauce, all GERD triggers. This version uses turkey breast meat—very lean—and egg whites to hold the loaf together. Onions are reduced to just a small amount, and tomatoes are gone altogether. All in all, a very simple and appetizing meal.

1½ pounds ground turkey breast meat, chilled
2 tablespoons chopped onions (as tolerated)
½ cup grated carrots
½ cup fresh bread crumbs
½ cup chopped fresh parsley
2 egg whites, lightly beaten
2 teaspoons ground cumin
1 teaspoon dried thyme, crumbled
2 tablespoons dried parsley flakes
1 tablespoon light soy sauce
1 teaspoon kosher salt

1. Preheat oven to 350°F. Spray a 9x5-inch loaf pan with nonstick cooking spray. Set aside.
2. Combine all loaf ingredients in a large bowl and mix with your hands. Transfer the turkey mixture into the prepared pan.
3. Cover with aluminum foil and bake for 30 minutes. Uncover, and cook about an hour more. Let stand for 10 minutes before removing from the pan and cutting into ½–¾-inch slices.

Makes 6 servings.

NUTRIENT ANALYSIS PER SERVING:

Calories (kcal) 120 ■ Protein (g) 21 ■ Carbohydrates (g) 4.4 ■ Fat (g) 1.5 ■ Saturated Fat (g) 0 ■ Sodium (mg) 484 ■ Cholesterol (mg) 33.7 ■ % Calories from Protein 72 ■ % Calories from Carbohydrates 15 ■ % Calories from Fat 11 ■ Total Dietary Fiber (g) 1

Grilled Marinated Lamb Chops with Cool Cucumber Relish

Grilled lamb chops are reminiscent of spring, though now tender young chops are available all year round. The cucumber relish is a perfect foil for the lamb, as well as chicken or fish if you desire. Grilling adds flavor to the lamb, which is good since we've eliminated trigger-ingredient onions and greatly reduced the wine and garlic in the marinade.

Lamb:
> 2 tablespoons olive oil
> 1/3 cup light soy sauce
> 1/2 cup dry white wine (as tolerated)
> 1/2 teaspoon chopped garlic (as tolerated)
> 1 teaspoon dried oregano
> 6 large loin lamb chops, visible fat removed

Relish:
> 3 cups fine chopped seedless or English cucumber
> 2 tablespoons rice vinegar (as tolerated)
> 1 tablespoon olive oil
> 2 tablespoons fresh chopped dill or 2 teaspoons dried dill
> 1/4 teaspoon salt, or to taste

1. Make the marinade: combine oil, soy sauce, wine, garlic (if using), and oregano in a small bowl and whisk well.
2. Arrange the lamb chops in a glass or ceramic dish and pour the marinade over the lamb chops and turn the chops to coat.
3. Cover the dish with plastic wrap and chill, turning two or three times for 4 hours up to two days.
4. Make relish: Combine all the relish ingredients in a glass or ceramic bowl and toss well (you may make this one day in advance).
5. Heat grill to medium high. Cook the lamb about 5 minutes per side for medium rare.
6. Serve chops hot with cucumber relish on the side.

Serves 6.

Nutrient Analysis Per Serving:

Calories (kcal) 328 ■ Protein (g) 37 ■ Carbohydrates (g) 3 ■ Fat (g) 17 ■ Saturated Fat (g) 5 ■ Sodium (mg) 410 ■ Cholesterol (mg) 122.7 ■ % Calories from Protein 46 ■ % Calories from Carbohydrates 4 ■ % Calories from Fat 47 ■ Total Dietary Fiber (g) .6

LIGHT SWEDISH MEATBALLS

No RESTRICTED-FOOD regime would normally ever include Swedish meatballs. They're full of fatty beef and swimming in sour cream. This version should be called Swedish-style meatballs because it removes the major GERD troublemakers without sacrificing flavor or texture. Turkey replaces ground beef, egg whites replace whole eggs, and fat-free sour cream is used instead of the real stuff. If dairy products don't agree with you, use nondairy sour cream. Serve these meatballs hot, spooned over cooked noodles.

MEATBALLS:
 1 cup plain bread crumbs
 2 egg whites
 ¼ teaspoon freshly grated nutmeg
 ½ teaspoon ground allspice
 1 teaspoon salt
 2 pounds ground turkey breast meat, chilled

 2 tablespoons olive oil
 3 tablespoons cornstarch
 ½ cup water
 3 cups beef stock or broth
 1 tablespoon Worcestershire sauce
 1 tablespoon fat-free sour cream
 ¼ cup chopped fresh dill
 Salt to taste

1. Preheat oven to 350°F.
2. Make meatballs: Combine crumbs, egg whites, nutmeg, allspice, salt, and turkey in a large bowl and mix with your hands.
3. Using wet hands, form turkey mixture into 1-inch balls. Chill until ready to use.
4. Heat oil in a large nonstick skillet over medium-high heat until hot.
5. Brown the meatballs on all sides and transfer them when browned to 9 × 13-inch baking dish.
6. Cover well with foil; bake in the preheated oven for 20 minutes.
7. Meanwhile, combine cornstarch and water in a small bowl and stir until smooth. Set aside.

8. In a large saucepan over medium-high heat, add the stock and Worcestershire sauce and bring to a boil.

9. Whisk in the cornstarch mixture and continue whisking until the liquid begins to thicken.

10. Remove from heat and gently whisk in the sour cream. Pour this mixture over the meatballs and stir well.

11. Keep warm until ready to serve.

MAKES 8–10 SERVINGS.

NUTRIENT ANALYSIS PER SERVING:

Calories (kcal) 160 ■ Protein (g) 19 ■ Carbohydrates (g) 10.7 ■ Fat (g) 4 ■ Saturated Fat (g) .5 ■ Sodium (mg) 447 ■ Cholesterol (mg) 27 ■ % Calories from Protein 48 ■ % Calories from Carbohydrates 27 ■ % Calories from Fat 24 ■ Total Dietary Fiber (g) .3

HEARTY BEEF STEW

SOMETIMES YOU JUST crave something homespun and comforting. If so, this is the stew for you. Most stews call for large amounts of onions and garlic; we've done away with the onions, and we've reduced the amount of garlic significantly. You may wish to reduce it even more or eliminate it entirely. The same is true of tomato paste, though the amount here is diluted by the large amounts of liquid. Most of the flavor of this stew comes from browning the meat first and then added vegetables and broth. If you're in a veggie mood, add peas and parsnips to the mix.

1½–2 pounds stew beef, cut into 1-inch pieces
½ cup flour for dredging
3 tablespoons olive oil
1 teaspoon minced garlic (as tolerated)
2 tablespoons tomato paste (as tolerated)
2 teaspoons dried thyme
2 teaspoons salt
1 tablespoon Worcestershire sauce
2 tablespoons dried parsley
8 cups low-sodium beef broth
1 cup chopped celery
2 cups 1-inch carrot chunks
2 cups 1-inch turnip chunks
2 bay leaves
6 cups 2-inch Idaho or russet potato chunks (peeled or unpeeled)

1. Dredge meat in flour and pat to remove extra flour.
2. Heat oil in a large pot over medium-high heat. Add meat and cook on all sides, until lightly browned.
3. Add the garlic (if using), tomato paste, thyme, salt, Worcestershire sauce, parsley, and broth to the pot and stir well.
4. Add the celery, carrots, turnips, bay leaves, and potatoes and stir again. Bring the liquid to a boil, then reduce heat to simmer. Cook the stew, uncovered, stirring occasionally, for 1 hour or until the meat is very tender.

5. Ladle the stew into shallow bowls or deep plates and serve with dark rye bread.

MAKES 8 LARGE SERVINGS.

NUTRIENT ANALYSIS PER SERVING:

Calories (kcal) 529 ■ Protein (g) 39.3 ■ Carbohydrates (g) 31 ■ Fat (g) 15.8 ■ Saturated Fat (g) 4.5 ■ Sodium (mg) 887 ■ Cholesterol (mg) 76 ■ % Calories from Protein 38 ■ % Calories from Carbohydrates 30 ■ % Calories from Fat 32 ■ Total Dietary Fiber (g) 3.8

GRILLED CHICKEN BREASTS WITH ORANGE HONEY SAUCE

THIS CHICKEN SOUNDS light and fruity—and it is. The sauce is almost invisible. It's pale in color, and its subtle flavors are simply delicious. Although the word "orange" will make some people apprehensive, the amount is small and, when cooked, is usually much less of a problem for GERD sufferers. Even without the orange, this chicken is extremely tasty.

CHICKEN:

8 boneless and skinless chicken breast halves (about 2½–3 pounds)
2 tablespoons vegetable oil
Kosher salt to taste
Sweet or mild paprika, to taste
Fresh minced parsley, garnish

SAUCE:

2 tablespoons olive oil
1 teaspoon minced garlic (as tolerated)
¼ cup honey
1 tablespoon grated orange peel (as tolerated)
1 cup fat-free chicken broth
¼ cup orange juice (as tolerated) or apple cider
1 tablespoon fresh tarragon, or 1 teaspoon dried
1 teaspoon ground cumin
1½ cups ½-inch diced zucchini

1. Heat grill to medium high.
2. Pound the chicken breasts with a meat mallet until about the same thickness throughout.
3. Brush chicken with vegetable oil and season it with salt and paprika to taste. Set aside.
4. Make the sauce: Heat olive oil in a large nonstick skillet over medium-high heat.
5. Add the garlic, if using, and sauté until softened, about 3 minutes.
6. Stir in honey, peel, broth, juice, tarragon, and cumin. Bring to a boil, reduce heat slightly and cook, stirring frequently, until the sauce is reduced and thickened to a syrup consistency.
7. Stir in zucchini and keep warm until ready to serve.

8. Meanwhile, grill chicken breasts until cooked through, about 4–5 minutes on each side.
9. Arrange the breasts on a platter and pour the sauce over. Sprinkle fresh-chopped parsley over and serve.

MAKES 8 SERVINGS.

NUTRIENT ANALYSIS PER SERVING:

Calories (kcal) 353 ■ Protein (g) 38.5 ■ Carbohydrates (g) 10.8 ■ Fat (g) 16.7 ■ Saturated Fat (g) 3.6 ■ Sodium (mg) 192 ■ Cholesterol (mg) 106 ■ % Calories from Protein 44 ■ % Calories from Carbohydrates 12 ■ % Calories from Fat 43 ■ Total Dietary Fiber (g) .5

PICNIC-GRILLED CHICKEN BREAD BOWLS

IMAGINE A MEAL all in one neat package. Buy bread bowls (usually used for serving soup) and scoop out the insides to use as containers for a mixed green salad with chicken. Then wrap up the bowl in a pretty napkin or new tea towel. Take these with you on a picnic or serve them at home for a fun lunch or dinner. Then eat the bowls. This is a low-fat and GERD-safe recipe that lets you add the amount of balsamic vinegar you can tolerate. If you can't tolerate vinegar at all, use a few drops of soy sauce instead. The juices from the cooked chicken act as dressing for the greens, too. For variety, use different herbs to season the chicken or substitute salmon fillet.

> *4 bread bowls (or small round bread loaves)*
> *1–1½ pounds boneless and skinless chicken breasts*
> *¼ cup apple cider or juice*
> *2 tablespoons olive oil*
> *1 teaspoon kosher salt*
> *1 tablespoon fresh rosemary or 1 teaspoon dried rosemary*
> *1 tablespoon fresh tarragon or 1 teaspoon dried tarragon*
> *¼ cup fresh minced parsley or 1 tablespoon dried*
> *1 red or yellow bell pepper*
> *4–6 cups mixed salad greens*
> *Olive oil, to taste*
> *Balsamic vinegar, to taste (as tolerated), or light soy sauce*

1. Prepare bowls: cut the tops of the bread bowls off horizontally about 1 inch from the top of the loaves (these will be the "lids" of the bowls). Use your fingers to pull the bread out from inside the loaf, leaving only a thick crust shell (this is the bowl). Set aside.
2. Pound the chicken slightly to a uniform thickness, or, if the breasts are very large, cut them in half, horizontally by pressing down slightly with your left hand and carefully slicing horizontally, beginning at the thickest part working toward the thinner part of each breast.
3. Place the pounded or sliced breasts in a medium bowl.
4. Add the cider, oil, salt, rosemary, tarragon, and parsley and toss well to coat the breasts. Cover the bowl with plastic wrap, chill and marinate for 30 minutes up to 3 hours.
5. Preheat grill to medium high.

6. Grill the pepper: Cut the bell pepper in half lengthwise and remove the stem and seeds. Place the pepper on the hot grill, skin side down. Grill for about 4–5 minutes, until lightly charred; then turn over to grill other side. When cooked through, remove from heat, cool slightly, and cut into thin strips.

7. Arrange the marinated chicken breasts on the grill and grill for 4–5 minutes on each side, until just cooked through (do not overcook).

8. Remove from heat and slice the chicken into strips.

9. Put the picnic together: Remove the "lid" from the bread bowls. Fill the bowls with salad greens. Divide the sliced chicken breasts among the bowls and replace tops.

10. Serve immediately, or wrap each lidded bread bowl in a large cloth napkin or clean new dishtowel. Tie together corners over the bread bowls or twist together the edges of the towels to make "bundles."

11. To eat, remove the napkins or towels from the bread bowls and use them as lapcloths or place mats. Remove the lids from the bread bowls and drizzle a little olive oil and balsamic vinegar, if using, over the salad and serve.

MAKES 4 SERVINGS.

NUTRIENT ANALYSIS PER SERVING:

Calories (kcal) 581 ■ Protein (g) 44 ■ Carbohydrates (g) 50.6 ■ Fat (g) 22 ■ Saturated Fat (g) 4.3 ■ Sodium (mg) 879 ■ Cholesterol (mg) 96 ■ % Calories from Protein 30 ■ % Calories from Carbohydrates 35 ■ % Calories from Fat 34 ■ Total Dietary Fiber (g) 7.6

CHICKEN WITH PEACHES AND WINE SAUCE

F RESH AND SUMMERY—ideal when peaches are at their peak. This is perfect served over cooked wild rice or your favorite pasta. You may also use apples, pears, nectarines, and plums (yes, plums). The alcohol in the wine evaporates while cooking, but still imparts a wonderful, complex flavor to the dish. Fat, onions, and garlic are reduced in this recipe and may be omitted if even small amounts cause great discomfort.

> *2–3 pounds boneless, skinless chicken breasts*
> *1 cup corn flour*
> *Kosher salt to taste*
> *¼ cup olive oil*
> *⅓ cup chopped onions (as tolerated)*
> *½ teaspoon minced fresh garlic (as tolerated)*
> *2 tablespoons dried parsley flakes*
> *4 large peaches, unpeeled, cut into thin wedges*
> *1 cup dry white wine*
> *3 cups chicken broth*
> *Sweet or mild paprika, to taste*

1. Pound chicken breasts to a uniform thickness, or cut, horizontally into thin slices.
2. Place corn flour in a small bowl.
3. Season the chicken to taste with salt and dredge the breasts in the corn flour. Set aside.
4. Heat oil until hot in a large nonstick skillet over medium high heat.
5. Add the floured breasts and sauté on both sides until lightly browned (you may have to cook the breasts in batches).
6. Remove the breasts to a dish as they're cooked and set aside.
7. Add the onions and garlic, if using, to the skillet (do not clean skillet first) and sauté them until softened, about 5 minutes, then sprinkle the parsley over.
8. Return the chicken breasts to the skillet and pour the wine and broth over (if your skillet isn't large enough, use two or transfer everything to a larger pot).
9. Arrange the peaches over the chicken.

10. Bring the liquid to a boil, reduce the heat, and cook until the liquid is reduced and slightly thickened. Adjust salt and serve the chicken with peaches and sauce spooned over and dusted with paprika.

MAKES 8 SERVINGS.

NUTRIENT ANALYSIS PER SERVING:

Calories (kcal) 346 ■ Protein (g) 31 ■ Carbohydrates (g) 21 ■ Fat (g) 14.5 ■ Saturated Fat (g) 3 ■ Sodium (mg) 318 ■ Cholesterol (mg) 77 ■ % Calories from Protein 35 ■ % Calories from Carbohydrates 24 ■ % Calories from Fat 38 ■ Total Dietary Fiber (g) 3.1

Eggplant and Spinach Lasagna

Aᴄʀᴇᴀᴍʏ, ᴠᴇɢᴇᴛᴀʀɪᴀɴ pasta dish that's the ultimate comfort food. This recipe makeover greatly reduces the amount of onions used and eliminates garlic and tomatoes, big GERD culprits. Because all the ingredients are low in fat, the pasta has a very light texture and flavor. If you'd like to make this dish with meat, add ½ pound cooked ground turkey breast or veal. This dish does include dairy products, which may not sit well with those who can't tolerate it.

> *9 strips dry lasagna noodles, any flavor, cooked al dente, according to package directions*

Fɪʟʟɪɴɢ:

> *2 1-pound whole eggplants*
> *2 packages frozen chopped spinach, thawed and drained very well*
> *½ cup chopped onions (as tolerated)*
> *2 cups shredded, lowfat mozzarella cheese*
> *2 cups lowfat or fat-free ricotta cheese*

Sᴀᴜᴄᴇ:

> *4 cups fat-free half-and-half*
> *6 tablespoons olive oil*
> *6 tablespoons flour*
> *Salt to taste*
> *½ teaspoon ground nutmeg*
> *1 cup fresh grated Parmesan cheese*

1. Preheat oven to 375°F. Spray a baking sheet with nonstick cooking spray.
2. Cut eggplant into thin (⅛-inch) circles and arrange on the baking sheet in a single layer.
3. Bake the eggplant for 15 minutes. Remove from oven to cool slightly.
4. Meanwhile, make the sauce. Heat half-and-half in a saucepan until boiling over high heat. Lower heat to simmer to keep the liquid hot.
5. In another small saucepan, heat olive oil over medium heat. Whisk in flour and cook, whisking constantly for 2 minutes.
6. Slowly whisk in the hot half-and-half until smooth.

7. Whisk in the salt to taste and nutmeg and cook the sauce, whisking constantly, until it's thickened slightly and smooth. Stir in the Parmesan cheese.
8. Spray a 9 × 13-inch baking pan with nonstick cooking spray.
9. Spoon ⅓ of the sauce into the baking dish and spread to cover the bottom.
10. Arrange 3 cooked lasagna noodles over the sauce.
11. Arrange half the eggplant slices over the pasta, overlapping the slices slightly.
12. Sprinkle ½ the mozzarella over the eggplant and dot with half the ricotta cheese.
13. Arrange another layer of lasagna noodles over the cheese.
14. Spread all the spinach over the pasta and sprinkle the onions over, if using.
15. Arrange remaining eggplant over the spinach and dot the eggplant with the remaining ricotta cheese.
16. Spoon another third of the sauce over the ricotta and top with remaining pasta. Sprinkle remaining mozzarella over the pasta and spoon remaining sauce over the cheese.
17. Bake the lasagna for 45 minutes, until browned and bubbly. Cool for 5 minutes before cutting into squares and serving.

MAKES 8 SERVINGS.

NUTRIENT ANALYSIS PER SERVING:

Calories (kcal) 406 ■ Protein (g) 31 ■ Carbohydrates (g) 42 ■ Fat (g) 20 ■ Saturated Fat (g) 7 ■ Sodium (mg) 611 ■ Cholesterol (mg) 34 ■ % Calories from Protein 27 ■ % Calories from Carbohydrates 36 ■ % Calories from Fat 38 ■ Total Dietary Fiber (g) 4

CREAMY SHRIMP AND PECAN PASTA

A DRESSY, CONTEMPORARY pasta dish with crunchy toasted pecans for fiber and low-fat broiled shrimp. The creamy sauce is very low in fat, but not apropos for those who cannot tolerate dairy products. Garlic, a major GERD trigger, is reduced considerably from other similar recipes. For variety, stir a few cups of fresh baby spinach leaves or chopped Swiss chard into the sauce before adding it to the pasta.

> 2 cups fat-free half-and-half
> 3 tablespoons olive oil plus 1 tablespoon olive oil
> 3 tablespoons flour
> Salt to taste
> 1/4 teaspoon ground nutmeg
> 1 1/2 cups chopped pecans, lightly toasted
> 1/2 teaspoon fresh minced garlic (as tolerated)
> 1 pound peeled and deveined large raw shrimp (about 30)
> 1 pound spinach fettuccine, cooked according to package directions
>   and drained but not rinsed
> 1 cup fresh grated Parmesan cheese

1. Heat half-and-half in a saucepan until boiling over high heat. Lower heat to simmer to keep the liquid hot.
2. In another small saucepan, heat 3 tablespoons of olive oil over medium heat. Whisk in flour and cook, whisking constantly for 2 minutes.
3. Slowly whisk in the hot half-and-half until smooth.
4. Whisk in the salt to taste and nutmeg and cook the sauce, whisking constantly, until it's thickened slightly and smooth.
5. Stir in the pecans and keep the sauce warm.
6. Heat remaining 1 tablespoon of olive oil and garlic, if using, in a large nonstick skillet over medium-high heat.
7. Add the shrimp and sauté for about 4 minutes, or until just cooked through (do not overcook or the shrimp will be rubbery). Season the shrimp with salt to taste.
8. Drain the pasta well, but do not rinse with water.
9. Transfer the pasta to a large bowl.

10. Add the shrimp and sauce and toss well. Serve immediately sprinkled with grated Parmesan cheese.

MAKES 8 SERVINGS.

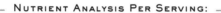

─── **NUTRIENT ANALYSIS PER SERVING:** ───

Calories (kcal) 529 ▪ Protein (g) 5.5 ▪ Carbohydrates (g) 48 ▪ Fat (g) 26 ▪ Saturated Fat (g) 4.5 ▪ Sodium (mg) 402 ▪ Cholesterol (mg) 174 ▪ % Calories from Protein 14 ▪ % Calories from Carbohydrates 28 ▪ % Calories from Fat 34 ▪ Total Dietary Fiber (g) 2.6

Buttermilk Oven-"Fried" Chicken

A REAL DOWN-HOME treat. Though not as decadent as the real thing—deep fried with extra-crispy skin—this version has much of that great taste without the ingredients, like large amounts of oil and garlic, which can incite GERD. Boneless and skinless breasts also make for easy eating and eliminate the fatty chicken skin.

6 large boneless and skinless chicken breasts (about 2 pounds)
2 cups buttermilk
4 tablespoons butter, melted
½ cup flour
½ cup cornmeal
1 teaspoon kosher salt
2 teaspoons paprika
1 teaspoon granulated garlic (as tolerated)

1. Soak chicken in milk in a large bowl. Cover with plastic wrap and chill for 30 minutes.
2. Spray a large baking dish or sheet well with nonstick cooking spray. Set aside.
3. Preheat oven to 400° F. Brush the butter over the bottom of the baking dish.
4. Mix flour, cornmeal, salt, paprika, and garlic (if using), together in a large zipper-style plastic bag.
5. Add one milk-soaked piece of chicken to the seasoned flour and shake well to dredge.
6. Place the dredged chicken breast in the baking dish and repeat with remaining chicken and flour mixture.
7. Bake for the chicken 10 minutes, turn it over, and bake an additional 10 minutes or until cooked through. Do not overcook.
8. Remove chicken from the oven and serve hot or at room temperature.

MAKES 6 SERVINGS.

NUTRIENT ANALYSIS PER SERVING:

Calories (kcal) 413 ■ Protein (g) 40 ■ Carbohydrates (g) 19.6 ■ Fat (g) 18 ■ Saturated Fat (g) 8 ■ Sodium (mg) 504 ■ Cholesterol (mg) 126 ■ % Calories from Protein 40 ■ % Calories from Carbohydrates 19 ■ % Calories from Fat 40 ■ Total Dietary Fiber (g) 1.3

Sautéed Mushroom Pasta

THIS IS A perfect recipe for mushroom lovers. For a less expensive, still delicious alternative, use all garden-variety button or white mushrooms. Be sure to clean the mushrooms well. For portabella and button mushrooms, use a damp cloth. For morels, cut them in half and soak. While mushrooms are often sautéed in GERD-triggering onions and garlic, they've been eliminated from this recipe. You may also substitute chicken broth for the wine.

> 8 fresh morel mushrooms or 8 dried morel mushrooms
> 3 tablespoons olive oil
> 12 ounces button mushrooms, sliced
> 2 large portabella mushroom caps, or equivalent, sliced thin
> ½ teaspoon kosher salt
> ½ cup white wine (as tolerated)
> ¼ cup fat-free evaporated milk or fat-free half-and-half
> ¼ cup fresh chopped parsley
> 1 pound dry fettuccine
> Fresh-grated Parmesan cheese, garnish

1. If using dried morel mushrooms, soak them in one cup of hot (not boiling) water for 30 minutes. Drain well and slice into rings. Set aside. If using fresh mushrooms, slice into rings and set aside.
2. Heat oil in a large nonstick skillet over medium-high heat.
3. Add all mushrooms and sauté for 5 minutes.
4. Add salt and wine and cook for 8 minutes. Stir in the milk and fresh parsley, and adjust salt to taste.
5. Cook fettuccine in a large pot of boiling water until al dente, according to package directions.
6. Drain well (do not rinse) and toss with the mushroom mixture.
7. Arrange on 8 plates and sprinkle with a bit of the grated cheese.

MAKES 8 SERVINGS.

NUTRIENT ANALYSIS PER SERVING:

Calories (kcal) 300 ■ Protein (g) 11 ■ Carbohydrates (g) 46 ■ Fat (g) 8 ■ Saturated Fat (g) 1.4 ■ Sodium (mg) 153 ■ Cholesterol (mg) 2 ■ % Calories from Protein 15 ■ % Calories from Carbohydrates 61 ■ % Calories from Fat 24 ■ Total Dietary Fiber (g) 2.3

GRILLED VEGETABLE SANDWICHES WITH ROASTED RED PEPPER MAYO

GRILLED VEGETABLES NEED very little embellishment. The essence of the fire is really enough, with a sprinkling of salt to bring out flavors. The roasted pepper mayo, however, is the jewel in the crown of this delicious sandwich. It does contain commercial mayonnaise that often includes GERD-instigating vinegar. The amount of vinegar is usually minute, so it rarely causes problems. Otherwise, it's a naturally reflux-friendly recipe. As a bonus, you can use the sauce for other things as well—as a salad dressing, vegetable dip, or with any beef, chicken, or fish as an instant condiment.

ROASTED RED PEPPER MAYO:
½ cup fat-free mayonnaise
1 roasted red pepper, homemade, canned or jarred, drained

VEGETABLES:
Olive oil, for brushing vegetables lightly
1 bell pepper, any color, cut in half lengthwise, stem and seeds removed
1 medium eggplant, unpeeled, cut lengthwise into ½-inch slices
3 carrots, peeled, cut in half lengthwise
3 zucchini cut in half lengthwise
12 large button or white mushrooms
Kosher salt to taste
Fresh French baguettes or 8 French rolls, for making sandwiches

1. Combine mayonnaise and pepper in the bowl of a food processor and process until smooth. Keep chilled until ready to use. (Makes 1 cup of sauce).
2. Preheat grill to medium high.
3. Brush the vegetables very lightly with the oil and grill them on a rack or over the grates of the hot grill, for 7–10 minutes on each side, or until cooked through. Hard vegetables, such as carrots, may take slightly longer.
4. Season the vegetables lightly with kosher salt. Cut the vegetables into smaller pieces.
5. Slice the baguettes into 6-inch lengths. Cut the pieces in half lengthwise but not all the way through, keeping a "hinge" at the bottom.

6. Fill the bread pieces with grilled vegetables.
7. Top each sandwich with a spoonful of roasted red pepper mayo and serve.

MAKES 8 SERVINGS.

NUTRIENT ANALYSIS PER SERVING:

Calories (kcal) 234 ■ Protein (g) 8 ■ Carbohydrates (g) 43 ■ Fat (g) 4 ■ Saturated Fat (g) .7 ■ Sodium (mg) 493 ■ Cholesterol (mg) 0 ■ % Calories from Protein 14 ■ % Calories from Carbohydrates 73 ■ % Calories from Fat 16 ■ Total Dietary Fiber (g) 5.8

APRICOT GINGER-GLAZED TURKEY BREAST

SWEET AND SAVORY flavors are paired in this very-low-in-fat recipe for turkey. We've added gingerroot and soy sauce to the mix for aroma and taste. For even less fat, remove the skin from the turkey just before brushing on the glaze.

>   1 3–5 pound whole bone-in turkey breast
>   1 can (15 ounces) fat-free chicken broth
>   2 tablespoons olive oil
>   1½ teaspoons kosher salt
>   1 cup apricot nectar
>   1 cup apricot preserves
>   1 tablespoon light soy sauce
>   2 tablespoons minced peeled fresh gingerroot
>   1 tablespoons dried parsley

1. Preheat oven to 400° F. Place turkey breast, skin-side up, in a small roasting pan.
2. Pour the broth around the turkey. Brush olive oil all over turkey and sprinkle with salt.
3. Roast the breast, uncovered for about 30 minutes. Reduce heat to 350° F and continue cooking for 30 minutes more, basting once or twice with the broth and drippings, as they collect.
4. Meanwhile, combine nectar, preserves, soy sauce, gingerroot, and parsley in a small saucepan over medium-high heat. Bring to a boil, reduce heat, and cook for 5 minutes, stirring occasionally.
5. Brush glaze over turkey. Continue to roast turkey, basting two or three times, for 30–40 minutes more, uncovered, until meat thermometer registers 180° F. or until juices run clear when the thickest part of the breast is pierced with a fork.
6. Transfer the breast to a platter and let stand 5 minutes before carving, or remove each breast half from the bones and cut into thin slices against the grain before serving it with pan juices spooned over.

MAKES 8–12 SERVINGS.

NUTRIENT ANALYSIS PER SERVING:

Calories (kcal) 334 ■ Protein (g) 42 ■ Carbohydrates (g) 31 ■ Fat (g) 5 ■ Saturated Fat (g) .8 ■ Sodium (mg) 404 ■ Cholesterol (mg) 115 ■ % Calories from Protein 50 ■ % Calories from Carbohydrates 37 ■ % Calories from Fat 13 ■ Total Dietary Fiber (g) .7

Grand Finale

ALMOST EVERYBODY HAS a sweet tooth (or a whole mouth full of them). Eating sweets is among the most difficult habits to alter. And giving them up all together is almost impossible.

The bad news is that chocolate doesn't have a place in these recipes—it's simply too aggravating. Citrus and peppermint, too, should be avoided or sharply limited. Most dessert recipes also contain one or more additional ingredients which are reflux triggers, especially butter, other fats, and dairy products. Often these are primary ingredients of many favorite desserts, from ice cream and cheesecake to cream pies and brownies.

All desserts call for sugar or other sweeteners. Some contain large amounts of sugar. As stated earlier in the book, sugar in baking and cooking acts like an acid. Large amounts of sugar, especially concentrated in icings, frostings, and many fillings, weaken the LES. If your sugar tolerance is low, limit your sweet desserts to a bite or two of your favorite gooey dessert or consume them earlier in the day when you will likely not be reclining.

The good news is that you can have your cake—or kuchen for that matter—and eat it, too. The key is using other fresh fruit in your desserts, limiting or replacing fats, and substituting egg whites for whole eggs. Intrinsically fat-free and very refreshing, fruits are wonderful cooked, because heat brings out their natural sweetness.

The following recipes are mostly fruity. Eat fruit desserts, too, in moderation for they can be acidic as well. Among the less acidic varieties of fruit are figs, dates, ripe bananas, persimmons, peaches, pears, guava, cherries, and certain melons, such as cantaloupe. Like all good things, however, the following desserts still include some foods we should eat less of, especially sweeteners and fats, and should be eaten with discretion.

Poached Pears

Poached pears are an extremely elegant dessert that's becoming more popular every day. Normally a pear is poached in a sugared wine broth, as it is here. The difference in this recipe is that the sugar is reduced significantly, and the amount of wine is cut significantly.

> *6 pears, firm yet ripe, with the stems intact*
> *Water, white wine, or both*
> *2 tablespoons sugar*
> *2 cinnamon sticks*

1. Find a pot or pan tall enough and large enough to hold all the pears standing up but not so big that they topple over.
2. Peel the pears, leaving the stems intact. Cut a thin slice from the bottom of the pears so that they can stand up without falling over. Place the pears in the appropriate pot, described above. Fill the pot with water, wine, or a combination of the two, until the liquid reaches more than halfway up the pears. Add the sugar and cinnamon sticks and bring the water to a boil over high heat.
3. Reduce heat to simmering and cover the pot. Cook the pears until they are softened and tender when a knife is inserted into the bottom half, but not so mushy that they begin to fall apart, about 40 minutes to an hour. Let cool completely in the pot and chill until ready to serve.
4. Serve pears in individual bowls with a little of the broth over the fruit.

Makes 6 servings.

Nutrient Analysis Per Serving:

Calories (kcal) 114 ■ Protein (g) .6 ■ Carbohydrates (g) 29 ■ Fat (g) 0.7 ■ Saturated Fat (g) 0 ■ Sodium (mg) 0 ■ Cholesterol (mg) 0 ■ % Calories from Protein 2 ■ % Calories from Carbohydrates 97 ■ % Calories from Fat 5 ■ Total Dietary Fiber (g) 4

BLUEBERRY MAPLE CRISP

BLUEBERRY PIE IS a perennial favorite each August when the crop is harvested and the price is low. Piecrusts, however, can be full of fat in the form of bits of cold butter, shortening, or lard. It's what makes crusts flaky and caloric. A crisp, on the other hand, is just a crumbled topping. Consequently, it may contain better fats, like canola oil, and needs not be particularly fatty. This recipe combines the summer flavor of blueberries with the ease a crustless dessert affords.

TOPPING:
½ cup unbleached flour
¼ cup chopped pecans
½ cup oats
⅓ cup packed brown sugar
1 teaspoon baking powder
1 teaspoon ground cinnamon (or more to taste)
⅓ cup canola oil (or other unsaturated oil)

BERRY MIXTURE:
5 cups fresh or frozen (thawed) blueberries
¼ cup maple syrup (as tolerated), or brown rice syrup
2 tablespoons brown sugar
¼ cup cornstarch

1. Preheat oven to 350°. Spray an 8-cup baking dish (such as a soufflé dish) with nonstick cooking spray.
2. Combine topping ingredients in the bowl of a food processor fitted with a metal blade and pulse until combined and crumbly. Set aside while you make the berry mixture.
3. Combine berry mixture ingredients in a large bowl and toss well. Transfer the berry mixture to the prepared baking dish and sprinkle the crumb topping evenly over the berries.

4. Bake for 30–40 minutes until the topping is golden and the berries are bubbling. Allow to cool before serving alone or with fat-free vanilla frozen yogurt.

Makes 8 servings.

Nutrient Analysis Per Serving:

Calories (kcal) 294 ■ Protein (g) 2.6 ■ Carbohydrates (g) 46 ■ Fat (g) 12 ■ Saturated Fat (g) 1 ■ Sodium (mg) 61 ■ Cholesterol (mg) 0 ■ % Calories from Protein 3 ■ % Calories from Carbohydrates 63 ■ % Calories from Fat 37 ■ Total Dietary Fiber (g) 3.7

STUFFED APPLE DUMPLINGS

APPLE DUMPLINGS ARE satisfying and homespun. Imagine an apple, stuffed with nuts and cinnamon wrapped in buttery pastry and baked. This version keeps all the good stuff—the apple, the nuts and sugar, albeit less than usual, but wraps the apple in fat-free phyllo dough instead of the high-fat pastry. A few drops of maple syrup before serving give the dough a shine that normally comes from brushing the pastry with egg yolks.

4 large golden delicious apples with stems
1 tablespoon sweet butter
2 tablespoons chopped pecans, lightly toasted
2 tablespoons brown sugar
½ teaspoon ground cinnamon
8 sheets frozen phyllo dough, thawed
2 tablespoons real maple syrup

1. Preheat oven to 350° F. Line a cookie or baking sheet with parchment or spray well with nonstick cooking spray.
2. Peel the apples, leaving the stems intact. Cut a thin slice from the bottom of the apples so that they can stand up without falling over. Core apples three-fourths of the way through from the bottom using a melon-baller. (Do not cut through the top.)
3. Holding the apple in your hand upside down, fill each apple cavity with a bit of butter, pecans, brown sugar, and ground cinnamon.
4. Place 2 phyllo sheets on a large cutting board or work surface (cover remaining dough with plastic wrap to keep from drying) and lightly spray the sheets with nonstick cooking spray.
5. Place 1 apple upside down in center of phyllo, pushing the stem through the dough. Wrap the dough around the apple and gather at the bottom of the apple.
6. Place in the apple-prepared pan, and spray the dough with nonstick cooking spray. Repeat with remaining apples.
7. Bake the apples for 30–40 minutes until the dough is golden. Remove from oven and cool at least 30 minutes before serving, drizzled with maple syrup.

MAKES 4 SERVINGS.

NUTRIENT ANALYSIS PER SERVING:

Calories (kcal) 325 ■ Protein (g) 3.3 ■ Carbohydrates (g) 63 ■ Fat (g) 8 ■ Saturated Fat (g) 2.7 ■ Sodium (mg) 188 ■ Cholesterol (mg) 8.2 ■ % Calories from Protein 4 ■ % Calories from Carbohydrates 73 ■ % Calories from Fat 23 ■ Total Dietary Fiber (g) 4.8

Fresh Strawberry Nests with Raspberry Sauce

KITAIF IS SHREDDED phyllo dough. It looks a little like angel hair pasta nests. You may have seen it in Middle-Eastern bakery goods. It's fat-free and looks quite fancy presented with fresh strawberries as in this recipe. The raspberry sauce is versatile—use it to top any number of desserts. This version has much less sugar than others and is fat-free.

1 pound kitaif (shredded phyllo dough)
Nonstick cooking spray
8 cups fresh strawberries

SAUCE:

2 cups fresh or frozen raspberries
¼ cup sugar
½ teaspoon vanilla or 3 tablespoons raspberry liqueur (as tolerated)

GARNISH:

Fat-free, nondairy whipped topping.

1. Preheat oven to 350° F.
2. Form as many loose small nests (about 3–4 inches in diameter), the size you like, from the kitaif and place each one on a baking sheet. Spray the nests with non-stick cooking spray and bake for 10–15 minutes until the nests are golden.
3. Make the sauce: Combine the raspberries and sugar in a medium saucepan over medium-high heat and cook until the sugar is dissolved in the cooking fruit juices. Stir in the vanilla and remove from heat. Allow the fruit to cool slightly before transferring the mixture to the bowl of a food processor and processing until smooth.
4. Place nests on individual dessert plates. Spoon the sliced strawberries over the nests and spoon ¼ cup of the raspberry sauce over each nest. Serve immediately with 2 tablespoons of fresh whipped cream or whipped topping if desired and serve.

MAKES 12 OR MORE SERVINGS.

NUTRIENT ANALYSIS PER SERVING:

Calories (kcal) 183 ■ Protein (g) 3.4 ■ Carbohydrates (g) 36 ■ Fat (g) 2.7 ■ Saturated Fat (g) .5 ■ Sodium (mg) 189 ■ Cholesterol (mg) 0 ■ % Calories from Protein 8 ■ % Calories from Carbohydrates 79 ■ % Calories from Fat 13 ■ Total Dietary Fiber (g) 4.3

Thanksgiving Pumpkin Custard Cups

PUMPKIN PIE IS always made in a fat-filled, and caloric, pie shell. Most recipes also call for large amounts of sugar, whole evaporated milk, and whole eggs. This recipe offers the wonderful spicy flavor of traditional pumpkin pie without the bad stuff. Sugar is reduced significantly, egg whites replace whole eggs, and fat-free evaporated milk cuts calories to a bare minimum.

3 cups cooked pumpkin puree (you may use canned)
½ cup sugar
⅓ cup brown sugar
6 large egg whites
2½ cups skim evaporated milk
2 teaspoons vanilla extract
2 teaspoons ground cinnamon
1 teaspoon ground nutmeg
¼ teaspoon ground cloves

1. Preheat oven to 300° F.
2. Fill a baking dish (you may need two baking dishes for this), large enough to accommodate 12 small (up to 6 ounces) ramekins (do not put the ramekins in the baking dish). Add one inch of boiling water to the pan and place the pan in the oven while you prepare the custard.
3. Spray the ramekins with nonstick cooking spray. Set aside while you make the custard.
4. Combine all custard ingredients in the bowl of a food processor and process until smooth, about 30 seconds.
5. Carefully divide this mixture among the 12 ramekins. Place the ramekins in the water-filled baking dishes. Bake the custards for 30–40 minutes, until just set. Cool before serving, or chill, covered with plastic wrap, until ready to serve.

MAKES 12 SERVINGS.

NUTRIENT ANALYSIS PER SERVING:

Calories (kcal) 128 ■ Protein (g) 6.4 ■ Carbohydrates (g) 25 ■ Fat (g) 0 ■ Saturated Fat (g) 0 ■ Sodium (mg) 94 ■ Cholesterol (mg) 2 ■ % Calories from Protein 20 ■ % Calories from Carbohydrates 80 ■ % Calories from Fat 3 ■ Total Dietary Fiber (g) 2

ROASTED PEACHES WITH BASIL AND ALMONDS

AMERICANS DON'T NORMALLY think of roasting fruits for dessert. This unusual practice is actually not so unusual in Italy, where peaches and almonds are commonly paired and basil brings out the flavor of the peach. The recipe contains a small amount of balsamic vinegar and brown sugar, which give the peaches a sweet-and-sour flavor. The amounts are small, when divided among the eight peaches in the recipe.

8 peaches, unpeeled, halved and pitted
4 tablespoons light olive oil
1 cup fresh basil leaves (not packed)
½ cup slivered almonds, lightly toasted
¼ cup balsamic vinegar
½ cup brown sugar
1 teaspoon ground cinnamon

1. Preheat oven to 400° F. Spray a large baking dish with nonstick cooking spray.
2. Arrange the peaches cut side up in the baking dish. Drizzle the oil over the peaches (in the well left by the pit). Place a few basil leaves on top, and sprinkle the almonds over. Drizzle the vinegar over the peaches and sprinkle the sugar and cinnamon over the peaches.
3. Roast the peaches, uncovered, for 20 minutes. Remove from oven and cool.
4. Chill, covered with plastic wrap, until ready to serve, up to 2 days. Serve the peaches (2 halves per person) in a wine glass or dessert dish with juices drizzled over. Or serve with nonfat vanilla frozen yogurt, as tolerated.

MAKES 8 SERVINGS.

NUTRIENT ANALYSIS PER SERVING:

Calories (kcal) 140 ∎ Protein (g) 4 ∎ Carbohydrates (g) 2 ∎ Fat (g) 3.5 ∎ Saturated Fat (g) 0 ∎ Sodium (mg) 3 ∎ Cholesterol (mg) 0 ∎ % Calories from Protein 9 ∎ % Calories from Carbohydrates 8 ∎ % Calories from Fat 29 ∎ Total Dietary Fiber (g) 1.5

DRIED CHERRY AND APRICOT KUCHEN

A KUCHEN IS very similar to a coffee cake. This version is an easy imitation because there's no yeast involved. It's also less caloric—with less fat and sugar—than the traditional version, which often includes cheese as an ingredient. That translates into less discomfort. For variety, try substituting fresh fruit or other dried fruits for the apricots and cherries.

    ⅓ cup chopped dried apricots
    ⅓ cup sweetened dried cherries
    1 cup boiling water
    2¼ cups flour
    1½ teaspoons baking powder
    ¾ teaspoon baking soda
    ¼ teaspoon salt
    1 cup skim milk
    ½ cup packed brown sugar
    ⅓ cup egg whites
    ¼ cup vegetable oil
    1½ teaspoons vanilla extract

TOPPING:
    ¼ cup finely chopped pecans
    2 tablespoons sugar
    1 teaspoon ground cinnamon

1. Place the apricots and cherries in a medium bowl and pour boiling water over. Allow the fruit to soak for 30 minutes. Drain well and set aside.
2. Place flour, baking powder, baking soda, and salt in a large bowl. Stir or whisk well to combine.
3. Preheat oven to 375° F. Spray a 9- or 10-inch springform pan well with nonstick cooking spray.
4. Place the drained apricots and cherries in large bowl. Add the milk, brown sugar, egg whites, vegetable oil, and vanilla. Stir or beat well. Fold in the flour mixture until just combined. Transfer the batter to the prepared pan.
5. Combine the topping ingredients in a small bowl and sprinkle over the kuchen batter.

6. Bake for 40 minutes or until a toothpick inserted into the cake comes out clean.
7. Cool completely before running a knife around the collar of the pan and loosening the sides. Cut into wedges and serve.

MAKES 12 SERVINGS.

NUTRIENT ANALYSIS PER SERVING:

Calories (kcal) 218 ■ Protein (g) 4 ■ Carbohydrates (g) 36 ■ Fat (g) 6 ■ Saturated Fat (g) .7 ■ Sodium (mg) 202 ■ Cholesterol (mg) .7 ■ % Calories from Protein 8 ■ % Calories from Carbohydrates 66 ■ % Calories from Fat 26 ■ Total Dietary Fiber (g) 1.4

Gingered Apple, Pear, Plum, and Almond Compote

COMPOTES ARE A wonderful way to serve fruit. Essentially the fruit is stewed in sugar syrup with cinnamon and cloves. This recipe uses fresh fruits with the addition of fresh gingerroot, which helps keep the LES closed.

> *4 cups peeled Granny Smith apples, cut into 1-inch chunks*
> *4 cups peeled ripe but firm pears (any variety),*
>   *cut into 1-inch chunks*
> *4 cups sliced plums (any variety), unpeeled*
> *1½ cups whole blanched, peeled almonds*
> *8 cups water or white wine, or combination*
> *½ cup honey*
> *6 cloves*
> *1 teaspoon vanilla extract*
> *1 teaspoon ground cinnamon*
> *1 inch unpeeled fresh gingerroot, sliced*

1. Combine all ingredients in a large pot over medium-high heat.
2. Bring the liquid to a boil, reduce heat, cover with a tight-fitting lid, and cook for 30 minutes.
3. Remove lid and continue cooking for another 30 minutes, until the syrup is reduced somewhat and the fruit is very tender.
4. Cool and store the compote in a nonreactive container, covered, in the refrigerator until ready to serve. Serve the compote in a large bowl or in individual dessert cups.

MAKES 12 SERVINGS.

NUTRIENT ANALYSIS PER SERVING:

Calories (kcal) 250 ■ Protein (g) 5 ■ Carbohydrates (g) 36 ■ Fat (g) 10.7 ■ Saturated Fat (g) 1 ■ Sodium (mg) 2 ■ Cholesterol (mg) 0 ■ % Calories from Protein 8 ■ % Calories from Carbohydrates 58 ■ % Calories from Fat 39 ■ Total Dietary Fiber (g) 6

CHEWY OATMEAL CRANBERRY COOKIES

COOKIES GENERALLY INCLUDE flour, butter, sugar, and, often, eggs. This recipe uses all these same ingredients, but in significantly smaller quantities and without egg yolks. Applesauce adds moistness that normally comes from fat, and the dried fruit and oatmeal make these cookies extra chewy.

1½ cups flour
1½ cups oats (not quick or instant oats)
1 teaspoon baking soda
1 teaspoon ground cinnamon
¼ teaspoon salt
¾ cup brown sugar
2 tablespoons butter, softened
1 teaspoon vanilla extract
½ cup unsweetened applesauce
2 large egg whites
1 cup sweetened dried cranberries

1. Preheat oven to 350° F. Line a baking sheet with parchment or spray well with nonstick cooking spray.
2. Combine flour, oats, baking soda, cinnamon, and salt in a medium bowl and stir or whisk well to combine. Set aside.
3. Using an electric mixer, cream together the sugar and butter in a large bowl. Stir in the vanilla, applesauce, and egg whites. Add the flour mixture and stir until just combined. Stir in the cranberries.
4. Drop large tablespoonfuls of the cookie batter onto the prepared baking sheet, 2 inches apart, spreading the batter with a spoon slightly.
5. Bake for 10 minutes. Cool before removing from the baking sheet. Do not stack the cookies on top of one another as they are soft and may stick together.

MAKES 3 DOZEN COOKIES.

NUTRIENT ANALYSIS PER SERVING:

Calories (kcal) 72 ■ Protein (g) 1 ■ Carbohydrates (g) 14 ■ Fat (g) 1 ■ Saturated Fat (g) 0.5 ■ Sodium (mg) 63 ■ Cholesterol (mg) 2 ■ % Calories from Protein 7 ■ % Calories from Carbohydrates 80 ■ % Calories from Fat 13 ■ Total Dietary Fiber (g) 1

BANANA CUPCAKES
WITH CREAM-CHEESE FROSTING

THIS RECIPE IS light, yet satisfying. Bananas are creamy and a good substitute for fat, adding texture without calories. Egg whites are fat-free; fat-free sour cream and cream cheese add even more creaminess to the batter and richness to the frosting. There's still sugar and butter in the recipe. Though amounts are reduced, these cupcakes should be eaten in moderation.

CUPCAKES:
1 cup flour
½ teaspoon baking soda
¼ teaspoon salt
½ teaspoon ground cinnamon
¾ cup granulated sugar
4 tablespoons butter, softened
1 teaspoon vanilla extract
½ cup mashed ripe banana
4 large egg whites
¼ cup fat-free sour cream

FROSTING:
1½ cups powdered sugar
8 ounces fat-free cream cheese, softened
1 teaspoon vanilla extract

1. Preheat oven to 350° F. Spray a 12-cup muffin tin well with nonstick cooking spray. Set aside.
2. Place flour, baking soda, salt, and cinnamon in a small bowl. Stir or whisk well to combine. Set aside.
3. Using an electric mixer, cream together the sugar and butter in a large bowl. Beat in the vanilla and the mashed banana. Add the egg whites and beat well.
4. Stir in half the flour mixture and the sour cream and then the remaining flour mixture until just combined.
5. Spoon the batter into prepared 12 muffin cups and bake for 25–40 minutes until a toothpick inserted in the center comes out clean.

6. Remove from oven and cool for 15 minutes before removing the cupcakes from the pan. Cool the cupcakes completely before frosting them or the frosting will melt.

7. Make the frosting: Beat all the frosting ingredients in a medium bowl until creamy. Spread the frosting thinly over the cupcakes using a spatula or knife.

MAKES 12 CUPCAKES.

NUTRIENT ANALYSIS PER SERVING:

Calories (kcal) 220 ■ Protein (g) 5 ■ Carbohydrates (g) 40 ■ Fat (g) 4.2 ■ Saturated Fat (g) 2.5 ■ Sodium (mg) 257 ■ Cholesterol (mg) 13.4 ■ % Calories from Protein 9 ■ % Calories from Carbohydrates 73 ■ % Calories from Fat 17 ■ Total Dietary Fiber (g) .5

DATE-WALNUT BARS

DATES AND WALNUTS are very low in acid. Combined in this recipe that removes much of the fat that's normally associated with pastry, they create an easy to make dessert that's made safer for GERD sufferers.

1 cup flour
½ teaspoon baking soda
¼ teaspoon salt
½ teaspoon cinnamon
¼ teaspoon freshly grated nutmeg
5 tablespoons butter, softened
½ cup sugar
4 large egg whites, lightly beaten
1 cup chopped dates
½ cup chopped walnuts
¼ cup golden raisins
Confectioners' sugar for dusting

1. Preheat oven to 350° F. Spray an 8 x 8–inch baking dish or pan well with non-stick cooking spray.
2. Combine flour, baking soda, salt, cinnamon, and nutmeg in a medium bowl and stir well with a fork. Set aside.
3. Use an electric mixer to cream together the butter and sugar until fluffy.
4. Add the egg whites, a little at a time, mixing well after each addition.
5. Add the flour mixture, dates, walnuts, and raisins, and mix until just combined.
6. Spread the mixture in the prepared baking dish and bake for 40 minutes.
7. Cool and cut into 1 x 2–inch bars. Remove the bars from the pan and arrange on a serving dish.
8. Just before serving, sprinkle with confectioners' sugar and serve.

MAKES 32 BARS.

NUTRIENT ANALYSIS PER SERVING:

Calories (kcal) 78 ■ Protein (g) 1.3 ■ Carbohydrates (g) 12 ■ Fat (g) 3 ■ Saturated Fat (g) 1.3 ■ Sodium (mg) 65 ■ Cholesterol (mg) 5 ■ % Calories from Protein 7 ■ % Calories from Carbohydrates 61 ■ % Calories from Fat 36 ■ Total Dietary Fiber (g) .7

Brunch Table

Breakfast is the easiest meal of the day for those with GERD. It's easy to pick a high-fiber hot or cold cereal that's low in fat and satisfying as well. Those who tolerate dairy products can add skim milk and many different types of fruit for an instant meal. Eggs are easy as well. There are egg-substitute products on the market, and egg white omelets are available at most restaurants these days. Sometimes, however, you crave something a little different or special.

Take weekends, for instance. Weekend mornings beg for brunch. You're often in no hurry to wake up, so that casual, even slow, preparation allows time for special foods not normally prepared during the week. Here's where potential problems arise. Many baked goods such as muffins and biscuits call for butter or oil and sugar, adding calories and fat. For GERD sufferers trying to lose or maintain weight, these are usually among the first foods eliminated from the acceptable-foods list.

Also removed from this list are spicy or fatty breakfast meats such as sausage and bacon, mainstays of what's know as the big American breakfast.

The good news is that you can have many of the foods you crave, as long as they don't contain excessive amounts of the trigger foods that cause reflux. All that's really needed are a few recipe makeovers to bring back most of the foods you love.

The following recipes may contain some ingredients you wish to avoid. The offensive ingredients, however, are reduced considerably, and, as part of the recipe as a whole, often minute when divided by the number of servings.

BARLEY FLOUR-DRIED BLUEBERRY BISCUITS

THESE ARE EARTHY, satisfying egg-less biscuits that are great for breakfast, spread with a little honey, jam, or lowfat butter. You can make the biscuits completely nondairy by substituting margarine or vegetable oil for the butter, and apple juice for the skim milk.

> 1¼ cups flour
> 1¼ cups barley flour (available at health food stores)
> 1 tablespoon sugar
> 1½ teaspoons baking powder
> ½ teaspoon baking soda
> 1 teaspoon salt
> ½ teaspoon ground cinnamon
> 1 cup skim milk
> 4 tablespoons butter, melted
> 1 cup dried blueberries

1. Preheat oven to 425° F. Spray a baking sheet with nonstick cooking spray or line with parchment.
2. Combine flours, sugar, baking powder, baking soda, salt, and cinnamon in a large bowl. Stir well to combine.
3. Stir in the milk until just combined.
4. Stir in butter and blueberries.
5. Use a tablespoon to drop about 24 large dollops of batter onto the prepared baking sheet. (Use the back of the spoon to shape the mounds neatly.)
6. Bake for 15 minutes until golden. Serve warm.

MAKES 24 BISCUITS.

NUTRIENT ANALYSIS PER SERVING:

Calories (kcal) 87 ∎ Protein (g) 1.6 ∎ Carbohydrates (g) 15.5 ∎ Fat (g) 2 ∎ Saturated Fat (g) 1.3 ∎ Sodium (mg) 175 ∎ Cholesterol (mg) 5.6 ∎ % Calories from Protein 8 ∎ % Calories from Carbohydrates 71 ∎ % Calories from Fat 23 ∎ Total Dietary Fiber (g) .7

Jeweled Granola

Many store-bought granolas are fat-and-calorie disasters. They're also quite pricey. This recipe is luxurious, jeweled with three types of dried fruits. Many people like granola served with nonfat vanilla yogurt spooned over instead of milk. If you can't tolerate dairy products, this granola is also good as a topping for fresh fruit or eaten out of hand, as a snack.

1 egg white, lightly beaten
2 tablespoons honey
¾ cup oats (not quick)
4 cups bran flake cereal
½ cup chopped pecans
¼ cup sunflower seeds
¼ cup sweetened dried blueberries
¼ cup sweetened dried cranberries or cherries
¼ cup golden raisins

1. Preheat oven to 325° F. Spray a baking sheet with nonstick cooking spray. Set aside.
2. Stir together the egg white and honey in a large bowl. Add the oats, wheat flakes, pecans, and sunflower seeds. Toss well to coat.
3. Spread this mixture over the prepared pan and bake for 20 minutes.
4. Remove from oven and let cool completely before breaking up the mixture with your fingers.
5. Toss in the dried fruits and store the granola in a zipper-style plastic bag or airtight container.

Makes about 6–7 cups of granola, or 10 servings.

Nutrient Analysis Per Serving:

Calories (kcal) 189 ■ Protein (g) 4.2 ■ Carbohydrates (g) 31 ■ Fat (g) 6 ■ Saturated Fat (g) .6 ■ Sodium (mg) 113 ■ Cholesterol (mg) 0 ■ % Calories from Protein 9 ■ % Calories from Carbohydrates 67 ■ % Calories from Fat 29 ■ Total Dietary Fiber (g) 3.5

BAKED GLAZED PINEAPPLE

CITRUS FRUITS MAKE up a substantial part of many breakfast meals. Since citrus is a great reflux inciter, it's necessary to look to other fruits. Pineapple, while acidic, is less so than citrus, so not as offensive, especially in small amounts. Alone, pineapple is certainly delicious. Glazed with brown sugar and a little real maple syrup, it's sublime. This recipe works well with other fruits, too. Experiment with different fruits to make a glazed warm fruit salad.

1 large fresh pineapple, peeled, cored, and cut into 1-inch chunks
½ teaspoon ground cinnamon
¼ cup brown sugar
¼ cup maple syrup

1. Preheat oven to 350° F. Spray a baking pan with nonstick cooking spray. Set aside.
2. Combine pineapple chunks, cinnamon, brown sugar, and maple syrup. Toss well and spread over the prepared baking sheet.
3. Bake for 30 minutes, turning once or twice. Serve warm, alone, or over pancakes or waffles as a topping.

MAKES 8 SERVINGS.

NUTRIENT ANALYSIS PER SERVING:

Calories (kcal) 55 ▪ Protein (g) .2 ▪ Carbohydrates (g) 14 ▪ Fat (g) 0 ▪ Saturated Fat (g) 0 ▪ Sodium (mg) 3.3 ▪ Cholesterol (mg) 0 ▪ % Calories from Protein 2 ▪ % Calories from Carbohydrates 94 ▪ % Calories from Fat 4 ▪ Total Dietary Fiber (g) .8

OVEN-BAKED POTATO PANCAKES

P OTATO PANCAKES, ALSO known as "latkes," are a perfect side dish or lower-fat alternative to hash browns. This recipe is even better for you, because the pancakes are baked instead of fried. That translates into less fat and calories for those looking to reduce both. While onions add flavor to the pancakes, you may choose to leave them out.

> *3 pounds potatoes (preferably Yukon gold)*
> *¼ cup minced onion*
> *⅓ cup flour*
> *½ teaspoon baking powder*
> *1 cup egg substitute, or 2 whole eggs plus 4 egg whites*
> *3 tablespoons chopped parsley*
> *1 teaspoon salt*
> *2–3 tablespoons canola oil*
> *1 cup nonfat or lowfat sour cream for serving, optional*
> *1 cup unsweetened applesauce, garnish*

1. Place a large nonstick baking sheet in the oven and preheat to 450° F.
2. Peel the potatoes and onion and coarsely grate both in a food processor fitted with a shredding disk or on a box grater. Grab handfuls of the grated vegetables and squeeze tightly to wring out as much liquid as possible.
3. Transfer the grated potatoes and onion to a mixing bowl and stir in the flour, baking powder, egg substitute, parsley, and salt.
4. Remove the baking sheet from the oven and spread the oil over the hot baking sheet. (Note: If working with a small baking sheet, you may need more oil.)
5. Spoon small mounds of potato mixture onto the baking sheet to form 2½-inch pancakes, leaving ½ inch of space between each pancake.
6. Bake the pancakes until golden brown, 6 to 8 minutes per side, turning once with a spatula. (When you turn the pancakes, try to flip them onto spots on the baking sheet that still have oil.)
7. Transfer the hot pancakes to plates or a platter and serve at once with sour cream and/or applesauce.

MAKES 50 TO 60 2-INCH PANCAKES, WHICH WILL SERVE 8 TO 10.

NUTRIENT ANALYSIS PER SERVING:

Calories (kcal) 251 ■ Protein (g) 8.4 ■ Carbohydrates (g) 44.5 ■ Fat (g) 4.4 ■ Saturated Fat (g) .3 ■ Sodium (mg) 181 ■ Cholesterol (mg) 0 ■ % Calories from Protein 13 ■ % Calories from Carbohydrates 71 ■ % Calories from Fat 16 ■ Total Dietary Fiber (g) 3

Oven-Baked Sausage Patties

Store-bought sausage is usually full of fat (up to half of some sausage patties are fat), sodium, and preservatives. They're also spicy—too spicy for most people with GERD. This lean version has just a little olive oil and is oven baked. Although it'll never be "regular" sausage, in texture or taste, you won't suffer eating these.

> 1 pound lean ground pork, chilled
> 3 tablespoons olive oil
> 1/2 teaspoon salt
> 1 teaspoon dried, crumbled sage
> 1/2 teaspoon dried thyme

1. Preheat oven to 400° F. Spray a baking sheet with nonstick cooking spray. Set aside.
2. Combine all ingredients in a medium bowl and mix well with your hands.
3. Using wet hands, form 1/4-cup portions of the mixture into small, flattened patties.
4. Place the patties on the prepared baking sheet and bake, turning once, until browned on each side, about 8–10 minutes.

Makes 8 servings.

Nutrient Analysis Per Serving:

Calories (kcal) 146 ∎ Protein (g) 10 ∎ Carbohydrates (g) 0 ∎ Fat (g) 11.6 ∎ Saturated Fat (g) 3.3 ∎ Sodium (mg) 173 ∎ Cholesterol (mg) 32 ∎ % Calories from Protein 27 ∎ % Calories from Carbohydrates 0 ∎ % Calories from Fat 71 ∎ Total Dietary Fiber (g) 0

Sweet Corn Pudding

H OT AND CREAMY, this dish is like a sweet cornmeal mush, which some call Indian pudding. It's a great side or dessert, when you feel like something homey and comforting. Lightly spiced, this version is fat-free, eliminating the butter and whole milk that's normally used in this recipe.

½ cup yellow cornmeal
4 cups skim milk
⅔ cup brown sugar
1 teaspoon ground cinnamon
1 teaspoon ground ginger
½ teaspoon ground nutmeg
1 teaspoon salt
1 cup frozen corn, thawed
⅓ cup molasses
1 cup nonfat evaporated milk

1. Preheat oven to 275° F. Spray a 2-quart glass or ceramic baking dish with non-stick cooking spray. Set aside.
2. Combine cornmeal and 1 cup of milk in a large saucepan over medium heat and stir well.
3. Add remaining milk and cook, stirring, until the milk is just about to boil (do not let boil). Reduce heat to medium and continue to cook, stirring, for about 5–10 minutes, until the mixture is thickened and smooth.
4. Remove from heat and stir in the cinnamon, ginger, nutmeg, salt, corn, molasses, and evaporated milk.
5. Transfer the mixture to the prepared baking dish and bake, uncovered, for 1½ to 2 hours. Cool slightly and serve warm.

MAKES 8 SERVINGS.

NUTRIENT ANALYSIS PER SERVING:

Calories (kcal) 223 ▪ Protein (g) 8 ▪ Carbohydrates (g) 48 ▪ Fat (g) .7 ▪ Saturated Fat (g) .3 ▪ Sodium (mg) 403 ▪ Cholesterol (mg) 3.3 ▪ % Calories from Protein 14 ▪ % Calories from Carbohydrates 86 ▪ % Calories from Fat 3 ▪ Total Dietary Fiber (g) 1.2

APPLE BUTTER

A WONDERFUL TOPPING for pancakes, waffles, toast, bagels, even frozen yogurt. Spread it on like jam, instead of high-fat butter or margarine.

> *3 cups apple cider*
> *2½ pounds apples (any variety), unpeeled, cored, and cut into chunks*
> *½ cup brown sugar*
> *½ teaspoon ground cinnamon*
> *⅛ teaspoon ground allspice*

1. Bring cider to a boil in a large saucepan over high heat.
2. Add the apple chunks, sugar, and spices and cook, stirring frequently, until the apples are mushy and the mixture is very thick.
3. Remove from heat and allow the mixture to cool completely before storing in a nonreactive container for up to one month in the refrigerator.

MAKES ABOUT 1½ CUPS.

NUTRIENT ANALYSIS PER SERVING:

Calories (kcal) 105 ■ Protein (g) 0.2 ■ Carbohydrates (g) 27 ■ Fat (g) 0.3 ■ Saturated Fat (g) 0 ■ Sodium (mg) 5.5 ■ Cholesterol (mg) 0 ■ % Calories from Protein 1 ■ % Calories from Carbohydrates 96 ■ % Calories from Fat 3 ■ Total Dietary Fiber (g) 2

PUFFY BAKED PANCAKE WITH FRESH BERRIES

THIS PANCAKE GROWS around the sides of the baking dish. As it grows, the sides "puff" out, giving the pancake its name. The sweet batter is usually made with whole eggs and lots of butter. This light version uses egg whites and light olive oil instead. And rather than topping the pancake with caloric maple syrup, fresh berries and a sprinkling of confectioners' sugar make it irresistible.

PANCAKE:

    12 large egg whites
    1½ cups milk or orange juice
    1 cup flour
    ¼ cup brown sugar
    ¼ cup sugar
    1 teaspoon vanilla extract
    3 tablespoons light olive oil
    ½ teaspoon cinnamon
    Confectioners' sugar
    5 cups mixed fresh berries
    Toasted pecans, walnuts, or almond slivers (optional)

1. Preheat oven to 425° F. Spray a large shallow baking dish (a 12-inch round dish or oval is best) thoroughly with nonstick cooking spray. Set aside.
2. Combine egg whites, milk, flour, brown sugar, sugar, vanilla, olive oil, and cinnamon in the pitcher of a blender of bowl of a food processor and blend or process until smooth, about 15 seconds.
3. Pour the mixture into the prepared dish and bake for 20 minutes until the sides rise and are puffy. Remove the pancake from the oven and cut into squares or wedges.
4. Serve hot, warm, or at room temperature. Sprinkle first with confectioners' sugar, then top with berries and nuts, if using.

MAKES 8 SERVINGS.

NUTRIENT ANALYSIS PER SERVING:

Calories (kcal) 251 ▪ Protein (g) 9.2 ▪ Carbohydrates (g) 39 ▪ Fat (g) 6.8 ▪ Saturated Fat (g) 0.9 ▪ Sodium (mg) 111 ▪ Cholesterol (mg) 0.8 ▪ % Calories from Protein 15 ▪ % Calories from Carbohydrates 62 ▪ % Calories from Fat 24 ▪ Total Dietary Fiber (g) 4

BREAKFAST POTATO PACKETS

GREAT FOR BREAKFAST and cleanup is a breeze. These potatoes are super-moist and steaming hot when you open the package. Great, too, if you want to cook these on the grill.

8 cups sliced new potatoes, unpeeled
1 chopped bell pepper, any color
4 tablespoons olive oil
Salt to taste
¼ cup fresh-chopped parsley or dill, garnish
2 cups diced very good quality ham, optional

1. Preheat oven to 400° F. Toss together all ingredients in a medium bowl.
2. Place a large (10-inch) length of foil on a work surface. Place another two sheets of foil on top, shiny side down. Spray the top layer of foil with nonstick cooking spray.
3. Transfer the potato mix to the foil. Bring sides of foil up around the potatoes and gather the sides up to seal. *Do not wrap tightly.*
4. Bake packet in the oven for 30–40 minutes, until the potatoes are cooked through, shaking the package every 10 minutes or so.
5. To serve, place the entire foil package on a serving dish and carefully open the top of the foil (so you don't burn your face or hands with the steam that's collected inside), and serve in the foil "bowl." You may also put the potatoes in a serving dish.

MAKES 8 SERVINGS.

NUTRIENT ANALYSIS PER SERVING:

Calories (kcal) 250 ▦ Protein (g) 11 ▦ Carbohydrates (g) 21.5 ▦ Fat (g) 10 ▦ Saturated Fat (g) 2 ▦ Sodium (mg) 538 ▦ Cholesterol (mg) 21 ▦ % Calories from Protein 17 ▦ % Calories from Carbohydrates 47 ▦ % Calories from Fat 36 ▦ Total Dietary Fiber (g) 3

SOUR-CREAM POUND CAKE

THIS IS A simple, dense pound cake. Old-fashioned pound cakes generally included a pound each of butter, flour, eggs, and sugar. This recipe retains the flavor and texture with a lot less sugar, eggs, and butter. That means less calories for those watching their weight. If you like more flavor, fold in 1 cup of chopped dried apricots or dried cherries to the batter, or a handful of poppy seeds, or sprinkle the batter with a little cinnamon and sugar before baking.

> *2 cups flour*
> *1 tablespoon baking powder*
> *¼ teaspoon salt*
> *½ cup sweet butter, softened*
> *1½ cups sugar*
> *4 egg whites, lightly beaten*
> *1½ cups fat-free sour cream*
> *2 teaspoons vanilla extract*

1. Preheat oven to 350° F. Spray a 10-inch bundt pan well with nonstick cooking spray. Set aside.
2. Combine flour, baking powder, and salt in a large bowl and stir well. Set aside.
3. In a large bowl and using an electric mixer, cream together the butter and sugar.
4. Add the egg whites and beat well.
5. Mix in the sour cream and vanilla.
6. Mix in the flour mixture.
7. Transfer the batter to the prepared pan and bake for 60–70 minutes, or until a toothpick inserted into the center comes out clean. Cool for 10 minutes before removing the cake from the pan.
8. Sprinkle the cake with powdered sugar and serve.

MAKES 12 OR MORE SERVINGS.

NUTRIENT ANALYSIS PER SERVING:

Calories (kcal) 290 ■ Protein (g) 5.4 ■ Carbohydrates (g) 48 ■ Fat (g) 8 ■ Saturated Fat (g) 5 ■ Sodium (mg) 192 ■ Cholesterol (mg) 22 ■ % Calories from Protein 7 ■ % Calories from Carbohydrates 66 ■ % Calories from Fat 26 ■ Total Dietary Fiber (g) 0.5

Spinach Brunch Soufflé

Savory soufflés start with a thick, white sauce, made with flour, butter, and milk. Egg yolks are added and egg whites folded into the mixture. This soufflé is no different except that the fat has been greatly reduced. This recipe calls for spinach, but broccoli, Swiss chard, pureed zucchini—really most anything can be put into a soufflé.

2½ cups fat-free evaporated milk
3 tablespoons olive oil
¼ cup flour
½ teaspoon salt
½ teaspoon ground nutmeg
½ cup minced onion
2 packages (10 ounces each) frozen chopped spinach, thawed,
    drained, and squeezed dry
1 cup fresh grated Parmesan cheese
8 large egg whites

1. Preheat oven to 400° F. Spray an 8-cup soufflé dish well with nonstick cooking spray. Set aside.
2. Heat milk in a saucepan until boiling over high heat. Lower heat to simmer to keep the liquid hot.
3. In another small saucepan, heat oil over medium heat. Whisk in flour and cook, whisking constantly for 2 minutes.
4. Slowly whisk in the hot milk until smooth.
5. Whisk in the salt and nutmeg and cook the sauce, whisking constantly, until it's thickened slightly and smooth.
6. Stir in the minced onion, spinach, and half the Parmesan cheese. Remove from heat to cool.
7. Using electric mixer, beat egg whites in large bowl until stiff but not dry. Fold ¼ of whites into the warm (not hot) spinach mixture. Fold in remaining whites. Transfer mixture to the prepared soufflé dish and sprinkle remaining cheese over.

8. Place soufflé in oven, reduce heat to 375° F., and bake until puffed and golden, about 35 minutes (the center of the soufflé should be set). Remove from oven and serve immediately.

MAKES 8 SERVINGS.

NUTRIENT ANALYSIS PER SERVING:

Calories (kcal) 181 ▪ Protein (g) 14 ▪ Carbohydrates (g) 11 ▪ Fat (g) 9 ▪ Saturated Fat (g) 3 ▪ Sodium (mg) 525 ▪ Cholesterol (mg) 11 ▪ % Calories from Protein 31 ▪ % Calories from Carbohydrates 25 ▪ % Calories from Fat 46 ▪ Total Dietary Fiber (g) 2.4 ▪ Total Dietary Fiber (g) 2.4

FRENCH TOAST WITH PECANS AND CARAMELIZED BANANAS

GOOD OLD-FASHIONED French toast is given a low-fat makeover and gets a facelift with sweetened bananas and toasted pecans. For more fiber, try a whole grain bread instead of the Italian.

3 ripe medium bananas, cut into ½-inch circles
2 tablespoons brown sugar
1 cup skim milk
½ teaspoon vanilla extract
½ teaspoon ground cinnamon
4 large egg whites
1 tablespoon butter
6 1-inch-thick slices Italian bread
¼ cup chopped pecans, lightly toasted
Confectioners' sugar for dusting French toast
½ cup pure maple syrup, warmed

1. Preheat oven to 350° F. Spray a glass or ceramic baking dish well with nonstick cooking spray.
2. Arrange bananas in the prepared baking dish and sprinkle with brown sugar.
3. Bake, uncovered, for 30 minutes, turning once during the baking.
4. Meanwhile, combine milk, vanilla, cinnamon, and egg whites in a medium bowl and whisk well.
5. Spray a large nonstick skillet well with nonstick cooking spray over medium-high heat. Melt a small amount of butter in the skillet and turn the skillet to distribute the melted butter.
6. Dip a bread slice in the milk and egg mixture, turning it over twice in the liquid. Add the dipped bread to the skillet. Repeat with remaining bread.
7. Cook the French toast, turning it once or twice until it is browned well on both sides, adding more butter and cooking spray as needed.
8. To serve the French toast, cut the breads in half, diagonally, and place 3 halves each on four dinner plates, overlapping them slightly.

9. Spoon the warm bananas over and sprinkle the pecans over. Sprinkle well with confectioners' sugar and drizzle the maple syrup over.

MAKES 4 SERVINGS.

─────────────── NUTRIENT ANALYSIS PER SERVING: ───────────────

Calories (kcal) 410 ▪ Protein (g) 11 ▪ Carbohydrates (g) 71 ▪ Fat (g) 9.6 ▪ Saturated Fat (g) 2.8 ▪ Sodium (mg) 430 ▪ Cholesterol (mg) 9.3 ▪ % Calories from Protein 11 ▪ % Calories from Carbohydrates 69 ▪ % Calories from Fat 21 ▪ Total Dietary Fiber (g) 2

Glossary

Abdominal cavity— The part of the body that contains the stomach, the small intestines, the colon or large intestines, the liver, the kidney, the pancreas, the spleen, the sexual organs, and the gall bladder.

Acetylcholine— A neurotransmitter that is released by the vagus nerve in response to the sensations of experiencing the look, the smell, and the taste of food.

Achalasia— A rare disorder in the intestines that is caused by lack of nerve response that would dictate normal swallowing patterns.

Acid reflux— Another term for gastroesophageal reflux disease (GERD).

Antacid— A type of medication that is used to lower the acidity of the stomach contents.

Antrum— The lowermost portion of the stomach.

Ascending colon— The portion of the colon between the cecum and the hepatic flexure, located on the right side of the body between the right hip and the ribs.

Anus— A sphincter that is attached to the rectum and through which fecal matter is eliminated from the body.

Bard procedure— Also known as the EndoCinch, this procedure involves the use of a stitching device attached to an endoscopic tool. The physician uses the device to place stitches in the LES and pull them together, forming a pleat and thus tightening the LES.

Barium XRay— This test involves the use of a contrast solution (barium) made of a smashed rock that is suspended in a solution. The patient swallows the solution and XRays are taken to reveal any motility issues or malformations in the upper gastrointestinal system. The type that is commonly used in GERD patients is known as the "barium swallow" or the "upper GI."

BARRETT'S ESOPHAGUS— A potentially precancerous condition of the esophagus that involves a change in cellular pattern in the mucosa that is usually related to long-standing GERD.

BERNSTEIN TEST— An older and not as widely used test for reflux, this method involves dripping hydrochloric acid alternately with saline into the stomach through a nasogastric tube and then measuring the patient's response.

BODY— The middle portion of the stomach.

CARDIAC ORIFICE— The point at which the stomach joins the esophagus and the location of the LES.

CECUM— A pocket-like formation at the entrance of the colon.

COLON— The large intestine.

COSTOCHONDRITIS— An inflammation of the rib cage that can be confused with the chest pain that some acid reflux patients experience.

DIAPHRAGM— A muscular-type membrane that separates the thoracic cavity from the abdominal cavity and is pierced by the esophagus.

DESCENDING COLON— The left-sided portion of the intestine that is located between the splenic flexure and the sigmoid colon. It is located between the ribs and left hip.

DUODENUM— The first loop of the small intestines that is about eight inches long.

DYSPHASIA— An uncoordinated or ineffective motion of the esophageal muscles that leads to an impaired ability to swallow.

DYSPLASIA— A change in normal cellular pattern that can herald the formation of cancer.

ENDOSCOPY— The practice of using a slim tool, the endoscope, that is used to examine the gastrointestinal tract and that is equipped with fiberoptic camera, cool lighting, and a biopsy snare.

ENZYMES— Chemicals that are produced in the liver, the pancreas, or the stomach and are used to break down the components of food for easier digestion.

EPITHELIAL CELLS— A type of cell found throughout the body. In the gastrointestinal system, they are found in the mucosa.

ESOPHAGEAL CANCER— A potentially fatal condition that results in many cases from years of damage due to reflux.

ESOPHAGEAL MANOMETRY— This test involves the use of special electrodes placed in the esophagus that track the movement of the muscles used during swallowing. It is generally used prior to surgery or when endoscopic tests turn up no visible sign of GERD-related damage to the mucosa.

Esophageogastroduodenoscopy (EGD)— Using an endoscopic tool, this test allows the physician to view the esophagus, stomach, and duodenum while securing biopsies of relevant tissues.

Esophagitis— An inflammation of the lining of the esophagus. In GERD, this is attributed to the erosive action of the acidic stomach contents on the sensitive esophageal mucosa.

Esophagus— A narrow, muscular tube that connects the pharynx to the stomach and aids in moving nutrients from the mouth into the stomach.

Fibrosis— Scar tissue.

Fundoplication— A surgical procedure, performed commonly with a variety of laparoscopic techniques, that involves wrapping the upper portion of the stomach partly or fully around the esophagus to tighten the LES.

Fundus— The uppermost part of the stomach.

Gas-bloat syndrome— A common side effect of surgical or endoscopic procedures that tighten the LES. Because digestive gasses and swallowed air can't escape as usual through the mouth due to the tightened sphincter, patients can feel bloated and experience a greater degree of flatulence following the surgery as the gasses and air must work through the intestines to the anus instead.

Gastrin— A hormone that is released by certain cells in the wall of the stomach.

Gastroesophageal reflux disease (GERD)— A condition in which gastric secretions splash past a weakened or incompetent LES into the esophagus or higher. GERD can cause erosive esophagitis, noncardiac chest pain, esophageal strictures, as well as a number of other esophageal and extraesophageal manifestations.

Gastroparesis— A condition caused by the paralysis of the stomach muscles. It can contribute to reflux symptoms due to the delayed emptying of the stomach that accompanies the condition.

Gastroplasty— A surgical procedure that involves slicing the gastric cardia in one direction, pinching the ends of the incisions together, and stitching the incision closed, thus lengthening the esophagus. The procedure is commonly used in combination with either a Belsey or Nissen fundoplication.

Heartburn— Another term for gastroesophageal reflux disease (GERD).

Helicobacter pylori— A type of bacteria that is believed to be the cause of ulcerations of the stomach and duodenum.

Hepatic flexure— The first turn of the colon between the ascending colon and the transverse colon. It takes its name from being located near the liver.

Hiatal hernia— A condition that is caused by a portion of the stomach forcing its way into the thoracic cavity. It is a common cause of reflux.

Histamine— A naturally occurring stimulant that is released during allergic responses as well as during digestion. In digestion, it prompts the release of hydrochloric acid.

Histamine H₂ blockers— A type of acid-reducing drug that blocks the uptake of histamines normally secreted during digestion, thereby cutting one of the chain reactions that results in the release of hydrochloric acid.

Hydrochloric acid— A caustic fluid produced in the lining of the stomach that combines with the enzyme pepsin to aid in digestion by chemically breaking down the components of nutrients.

Ileocecal valve— A muscular formation that joins the last loop of the small intestine (ileum) with the first turn of the large intestine (cecum).

Ileum— The last loop of the small intestines, about 12 feet long.

Jejunum— The second loop of the small intestines, approximately eight feet long.

Laparoscope— An endoscopic tool that is used with surgical attachments to examine the abdominal cavity and perform surgical functions.

Larynx— Located between the pharynx and the trachea, this organ supplies humans with voice. Aspirated acid can damage the larynx, causing a hoarse voice in some.

Lower esophageal sphincter (LES)— A muscular junction that connects the esophagus with the stomach. An incompetent LES contributes to reflux.

Lumen— The hollow part of an organ. In the GI system, the lumen generally is surrounded by the mucosa.

Mucosa— The innermost layer of the intestines.

Mucous— A clear, liquid secretion of the mucosa.

Muscularis mucosa— A layer of smooth muscle cells that surround the mucosa and submucosa. When contracting, this layer helps to move digested matter through the intestines.

Parietal cell— A type of cell located in the lining of the intestine that is prompted to manufacture and release hydrochloric acid during digestion.

Pepsin— An enzyme produced in the lining of the stomach that combines with hydrochloric acid to aid in digestion by chemically breaking down the components of nutrients.

Peristalsis— Intestinal movement used to propel digested matter forward, caused by contracting and relaxing of muscles in the intestinal wall.

pH scale— A rating system to rank objects according to acidity, neutrality, or alkalinity. The scale runs from zero to fourteen, with seven being neutral. A rating below seven is considered acidic, a rating above seven is considered alkaline.

Pharynx— Located between the esophagus and the oral and nasal cavities.

PROKINETIC AGENT– A type of medication that works to increase peristalsis, thereby reducing the amount of time that digested matter spends in the stomach.

PROTON PUMP INHIBITORS– A type of medication that travels through the bloodstream and bonds with the tiny proton pumps on the surface of the parietal cell to halt the production of hydrochloric acid.

PYLORUS– The muscular area located in the stomach's antrum portion. The pylorus opens to allow digested matter into the small intestine.

RECTUM– An elastic, muscular formation that is located between the sigmoid colon and the anus. This area acts to store fecal matter until it is ready to be eliminated.

REFLUX– Another term for gastroesophageal reflux disease (GERD).

SALIVATION– The act of producing saliva, a clear liquid that is secreted in the mouth and helps to clear the esophagus of excess acid.

SCLERODERMA– An autoimmune condition that causes the body to deposit collagen in the skin and in connective tissues. Many individuals with the disease will develop GERD, due to the buildup of scarred muscle tissue in the esophagus that impairs swallowing and is attributed to stricture formation.

SCINTIGRAPHY– This test is used to determine the transit time of foods through the stomach in certain patients who are suspected of having gastroparesis. The patient eats a food that is laced with a quickly dissipating radionuclitide and special photographs are taken with a gamma camera to track the food's progress through the stomach.

SIGMOID COLON– This S-shaped portion of the colon is located between the descending colon and the rectum.

SPECTROPHOTOMETER– This test is used in patients whose reflux may involve bilirubin as opposed to hydrochloric acid. The equipment used is similar to that which is used in the 24-hour ambulatory pH test, but the sensors are more sensitive to the bilirubin's higher pH.

SPHINCTER– A muscular formation that, when it constricts, reduces the size of the lumen.

SPLENIC FLEXURE– The turn in the colon that is located between the transverse colon and the descending colon. It is named for its location near the spleen.

STRETTA PROCEDURE– A procedure in which the LES is heated using radiofrequency waves, causing blood to coagulate at the site. After healing, this causes a thicker and tighter LES.

SUBMUCOSA– The layer of the intestinal wall between the mucosa and the muscularis mucosa.

STOMACH– A part of the gastrointestinal tract located between the esophagus and the duodenum, this organ is responsible for grinding food through chemical and mechanical activity to allow for later absorption by the small intestines.

THORACIC CAVITY– Located above the diaphragm in the chest area, this part of the body contains the lungs, the heart, and the esophagus.

TRACHEA– A hollow tube that opens in the pharynx and leads to the bronchea.

TRANSVERSE COLON– The only stretch of colon that is horizontal. It is located between the hepatic flexure and the splenic flexure.

24-HOUR AMBULATORY pH MONITORING– This test is commonly used prior to surgery as well as in patients in whom there is no visible sign of GERD-related damage in the esophagus. In the test, the patient wears a pH-sensitive monitor in the esophagus for one full day as the equipment regularly checks the acidity of the esophagus at various points.

VAGUS NERVE– A nerve that branches out to supply much of the upper gastrointestinal system, including the esophagus and the stomach.

VILLI– Little, finger-like projections found on the surface of the small intestinal mucosa. These projections allow for the absorption of nutrients.

ZOLLINGER-ELLISON SYNDROME– A very rare gastrointestinal condition that causes the formation of tumors in the stomach and pancreas as well as the formation of peptic ulcers. Additionally, the condition causes the parietal cells to secrete too much hydrochloric acid.

FOR FURTHER READING

Basic gastroesophageal reflux disease and digestion information

Berkson, D. Lindsey. *Healthy Digestion the Natural Way: Preventing and Healing Heartburn, Constipation, Gas, Diarrhea, Inflammatory Bowel and Gallbladder Diseases, Ulcers, Irritable Bowel Syndrome, Food Allergies, and More.* Hoboken, NJ: John Wiley & Sons, 2000.

Janowitz, Henry D. *Indigestion: Living Better with Upper Intestinal Problems from Heartburn to Ulcers and Gallstones.* New York: Oxford University Press, 1994.

Minocha, Anil, Christine Adamec. *How to Stop Heartburn: Simple Ways to Heal Heartburn and Acid Reflux.* New York: John Wiley & Sons, Inc., 2001.

Diet and nutrition

Janowitz, Henry D. *Good Food for Bad Stomachs: The Healthy Guide for Anyone Who's Ever Had an Upset Stomach.* New York: Oxford University Press, 1997.

In-depth reading about reflux

Freston, James W., ed. *Diseases of the Gastroesophageal Mucosa: The Acid Related Disorders.* Totowa, NJ: Humana Press, 2001.

Orlando, Roy C., ed. *Gastroesophageal Reflux Disease.* 1st ed. New York: Marcel Dekker, 2000.

Cooking and baking

Bluestein, Barry, Kevin Morrissey. *Guilt-Free Frying: All of Your Favorite Fried Foods with No Muss, No Fuss, and Almost No Fat!* New York: H. P. Books, 1999.

Mateljan, George, et al. *Baking Without the Fat.* Irwindale, CA: Health Valley Foods Company, 1994.

Rombauer, Irma S., et al. *The New Joy of Cooking.* New York: Scribner, 1997.

RESOURCES

Association of Gastrointestinal Motility Disorders, Inc.
11 North Street
Lexington, MA 02420
Phone: (781) 861-3874
Fax: (781) 861-7834
E-mail: *agmdinc@aol.com*
www.digestivemotility.org

***Digestive Health & Nutrition* magazine**
American Gastroenterological Association
7910 Woodmont Avenue, 7th Floor
Bethesda, MD 20814
(310) 654-2055
www.dhn-online.com

Heartburn-Help.com

International Foundation for Functional Gastrointestinal Disorders (IFFGD)
P.O. Box 170864
Milwaukee, WI 53217
Phone: 1-888-964-2001 or (414) 964-1799
Fax: (414) 964-7176
E-mail: ***iffgd@iffgd.org***
www.iffgd.org

International Foundation for Functional Gastrointestinal Disorders (IFFGD), Inc. Pediatric

158 Pleasant Street
North Andover, MA 01845
Phone: 1-800-394-2747 or (978) 685-4477
Fax: (978) 685-4488
E-mail: *aanastas@iffgd.org*
www.aboutkidsgi.org

National Center for Complementary and Alternative Medicine Clearinghouse
P.O. Box 8218
Silver Spring, MD 20892
(888) 644-6226
www.nccam.nih.gov

National Digestive Disease Information Clearinghouse
2 Information Way
Bethesda, MD 20892-3570
(800) 891-5389 or (301) 654-3810
E-mail: *nddic@infor.niddk.nih.gov*

Pediatric/Adolescent Gastroesophageal Reflux Association, Inc. (PAGER)
P.O. Box 1153
Germantown, MD 20875-1153
Phone: (301) 601-9541 (East Coast) or
(760) 747-5001 (West Coast)
Fax: (630) 982-6418
E-mail: *GERGROUP@aol.com*
www.reflux.org

Acknowledgments

I OWE A GREAT deal of thanks to Matthew Lore, my editor and publisher. Aside from green-lighting the project, Matthew helped to shape the manuscript in both major and subtle ways, making suggestions prior to the proposal and after it was finished. He is a fantastic editor, and I am truly blessed to work with him. Janis Donnaud, my agent, played a paramount role in helping me to fine-tune the proposal and in following through with the contract for it as well. In the months that followed, she also provided invaluable guidance and support, for which I am truly grateful. Sue McCloskey and Peter Jacoby, also at Marlowe & Company, kept me on target with gentle guidance and suggestions.

This book also would not have been possible without the kitchen wizardry of Annabel Cohen. Although at times my general nervousness regarding self-set deadlines bordered on nagging, she was more than willing to go along on this adventure with me, lending her deep reserve of culinary talent to the project. She is a fantastic sport, and I thank her for that. My father-in-law, Dr. Manuel Sklar, provided great assistance in the project by plying me with literally stacks of research papers as well as his thorough reading and correcting of each chapter. A gastroenterologist in practice for several decades, his insight and knowledge were just what this book needed. I also owe him one for writing the foreword.

My family remains my pillar of support. Joel and Jonah Sklar, my husband and son, respectively, encouraged me to dive into the project and continue to swim with it, frequently at the expense of the quality of their own meals. My mother, Kathryn

Davidson; my sister, Patrice Rink; my brother, Greg Davidson; and my sister-in-law, Megan Davidson, continued to nourish me through food and gossip every Friday lunch, not showing their disappointment too much when I had to skip the festivities to work on a chapter. My little brother, Eric Davidson, was kind enough to share his experiences and encourage me during the writing process, even as he was planning and celebrating his own wedding to Amy. My mother-in-law, Harriet Sklar, made helpful suggestions on the copy and on the recipes.

In particular, I must extend great thanks to all of those whom I have never met face-to-face but who shared their stories with me. Many of these individuals are from Heartburn-Help.com's message board, including the board's founder Robert Foster. Robert allowed me to post some of the recipes on the site and allow reader feedback, a big help initially in determining what kind of recipes people wanted. Robin David Taviner, a former heartburn sufferer and all-around mensch, plied me with information as well as humor breaks with his hilarious writing. Additionally, Sue Ann Spencer, Kathy Metzger, John Coffey, James Cribb, Marge Normille, Geary Wooten, Gilda Hauser, Sierra Donovan, Patti Kommel, and many others shared their stories with me to illustrate various points of the text. Their bravery in the face of at times life-altering pain is remarkable.

—*Jill Sklar*

Thanks to all my friends and family who have tasted, critiqued, and swallowed so many of my recipes all these years and who've been sometimes painfully honest about my not-so-successful attempts. An extra thank-you goes my daughter, Raquel, who often dined on GERD test foods without even knowing it and slept soundly while I tested recipes in the middle of the night. Special gratitude goes to Jill Sklar for the golden opportunity of contributing to this book.

—*Annabel Cohen*

INDEX

G

G cells, 17
gas-bloat syndrome, 71, 255
gassy vegetables, 49
gastrin, 17–18, 255
gastroesophageal reflux disease (GERD). *see* acid
    reflux
gastroparesis, 18, 255
gastroplasty, 255
GERD. *see* acid reflux
ginger, 79
Gingered Apple, Pear, Plum, and Almond
    Compote, 232
Granola, Jeweled, 239
Green Beans with Pecans and Warm Honeyed
    Apple Dressing, 143
Grilled Chicken Breasts with Orange Honey
    Sauce, 206–7
Grilled Marinated Flank Steak, 199
Grilled Marinated Lamb Chops with Cool
    Cucumber Relish, 201
Grilled Mustard-Based Shrimp Kebabs, 192
Grilled Vegetable Sandwiches with Roasted Red
    Pepper Mayo, 218–19
*Growth of Gastroenterologic Knowledge during the
    Twentieth Century* (Kirsner), 10
guided imagery, 82

H

heartburn, 19, 87, 255
    see also acid reflux
Hearty Beef Stew, 204–5
Hearty Fish Chowder in Bread Bowls, 126–27
heliobacter pylori, 31, 255
hepatic flexure, 18, 255
Herb and Olive Oil Roasted Green Beans,
    164
herbal remedies, 78–80
Herbed Oven Steak Fries, 167
hiatal hernia, 11, 22, 66, 95, 255
hiccupping, 20
histamine H2 blockers, 53, 55–57, 63, 90, 94,
    256
histamines, 17, 256
Hoisin Peanut Sauce, 113
hors d'oeuvres. *see* appetizers
Horseradish Mashed Yukon Gold Potatoes,
    171
hospital experience, 71–74
hydrochloric acid, 8, 256

I

ibuprofen, 62
ileocecal valve, 18, 256
ileum, 18, 256
inflammation, 19
International Foundation for Functional
    Gastrointestinal Disorders (IFFGD),
    261
intestine, 18
Israeli Couscous with Roasted Red Peppers and
    Chickpeas, 180–81

J

jejunum, 18, 256
Jeweled Granola, 239

K

ketoprofen, 62
Kirsner, Joseph, 10

L

lamb
    Grilled Marinated Lamb Chops with Cool
        Cucumber Relish, 201
    Slow-Cooked Lamb Chops with Oregano,
        198
lansoprazole, 58, 90
laparoscope, 67, 256
larynx, 20, 256
Lasagna, Eggplant and Spinach, 212–13
Layered Maple Sweet Potatoes with Pecans,
    183
legumes. *see* beans
Lentil Soup, 139
LES. *see* lower esophageal sphincter
licorice root, 79
lifestyle changes, 35–51
    changing diet, 46–51
    dressing sensibly, 43–44
    exercising, 41–43
    losing weight, 38–41
    during pregnancy, 87–88
    quitting smoking, 36–37
    reducing/eliminating alcohol, 37–38
    sleeping positions, 44–45
Light Swedish Meatballs, 202–3
Lind fundoplication, 68
linden, 80
lower esophageal sphincter (LES), 8, 20-24, 256
lumen, 16, 256

sugar, 49–50, 105, 221
Summer Rolls, 112–13
surgery, 65–76
    see also endoscopic procedures
    for children, 94–95
    diet tips following, 74–75
    experience of, 71–74
    fundoplication, 67–69, 72
    as last resort, 52
    questions to ask before, 75–76
    reasons for, 66–67
    recovery from, 73–74
    risks of, 70–71
    types of, 67–70
swallowing difficulties, 21
Sweet Corn Pudding, 243
Sweet Potatoes with Pecans, Layered Maple, 183
symptoms, 3–4, 9, 19–22

T

Tabouli Pasta Salad, 153
Tagamet, 56, 90, 94
tai chi, 83–84
Tapenade, 116
tela submucosa, 16
tests, 26–30
Thal fundoplication, 68
Thanksgiving Pumpkin Custard Cups, 228
thoracic cavity, 17, 258
Toupet fundoplication, 69
trachea, 21, 258
transverse colon, 18, 258
traveling, 50–51
treatment
    alternative, 77–84
    going without, 32–34
    medical, 52–64
    medications, 53–64
    during pregnancy, 87–88
    surgical, 65–76
tricyclic antidepressants, 24
trigger foods, 103–4
tuna
    Romaine Salad with Tuna, White Beans and
        Greek Olives, 148–49
    Seared Tuna with Raisins and Capers, 193
turkey
    Apricot Ginger-Glazed Turkey Breast, 220
    Light Swedish Meatballs, 202–3

Turkey and Wild Rice Soup, 132
Turkey "Meatloaf", 200
24-hour ambulatory pH monitoring, 29–30, 92,
    258

V

vagus, 16, 17
vagus nerve, 258
Vegetable Kebabs, 174
vegetables
    see also specific types
    Eight-Vegetable Minestrone, 128–29
    Grilled Vegetable Sandwiches with Roasted
        Red Pepper Mayo, 218–19
    Roasted Vegetable Soup, 125
    Seven Vegetable Moroccan-Style Couscous,
        196–97
    Vegetable Kebabs, 174
villi, 16, 258
vinegar, 50
voice changes, 21
vomiting, 20

W

Watercress Salad with Peaches and Warm Herb
    Dressing, Spinach and, 156–57
Watson fundoplication, 69
weight loss, 38–41, 104
Weight Watchers, 40
Wheat Berry Salad with Grilled Chicken and
    Peas, 152
Winter Squash Soup, 131

X

Xenical, 41

Y

Yams with Rosemary and Balsamic Vinegar,
    Roasted, 179
yoga, 83–84

Z

Zantac, 56–57, 90, 94
Zollinger-Ellison syndrome, 23, 32, 258
zucchini
    Seared Scallops with Carrots, Zucchini, and
        Parsley, 187
    Zucchini and Sun-Dried Tomato Crostini,
        117